# Aids to Paediatrics for Undergraduates

# Other titles in the Aids series

# Aids to Paediatrics for Undergraduates

**Alex Habel**
MB, ChB, MRCP (UK)
Consultant Paediatrician,
West Middlesex University
Hospital

CHURCHILL LIVINGSTONE
EDINBURGH LONDON MELBOURNE AND NEW YORK 1987

CHURCHILL LIVINGSTONE
Medical Division of Longman Group UK Limited

Distributed in the United States of America by
Churchill Livingstone Inc., 1560 Broadway, New
York, N. Y. 10036, and by associated companies,
branches and representatives throughout the
world.

First published 1987

ISBN 0 443 03217 3

British Library Cataloguing in Publication Data
Habel, Alex
    Aids to paediatrics for undergraduates.
    1. Pediatrics
    I. Title
    618. 92 RJ45

Library of Congress Cataloging in Publication Data
Habel, Alex.
    Aids to paediatrics for undergraduates.
    Includes index.
    1. Pediatrics – Outlines, syllabi, etc. I.Title
[DNLM: 1. Pediatrics – outlines. WS 18 H113ab]
RJ48.3.H33   1986     618.92    86–12917

Produced by Longman Singapore Publishers (Pte) Ltd.
Printed in Singapore

# Preface

In preparing this book for undergraduates I have been guided by my own impressions of the needs of today's students for a simple and practical approach to the physical examination of children, as well as the demands of the examiners.

As usual, lists are compiled in order of frequency and importance; the two are not mutually inclusive. An ordered approach, using 'first principles' where possible, will always help the candidate get to grips with a question, even without the benefit of a detailed knowledge of paediatrics. This book aims at consolidating that approach.

Students will be well served by *Essential Paediatrics* (1981) by D. Hull and D. I. Johnston (Churchill Livingstone). More comprehensive is *A Synopsis of Children's Diseases* (6th edition–1985) by J. Rendle-Short, O. P. Gray and J. A. Dodge (Wright). Standard textbooks are *Nelson's Textbook of Paediatrics* (12th edition–1983) by R. E. Behrman and V. C. Vaughan (Saunders) and Forfar and Arneil's *Textbook of Paediatrics* (3rd edition–1984) (Churchill Livingstone), which are good for general reference.

Thanks go to my teachers, the students. To my family and my colleagues, especially Peter Husband, I owe a debt for their encouragement and forbearance.

Isleworth, 1987

A. H.

# Contents

# Introduction

**GENERAL HINTS ON PHYSICAL EXAMINATION**

## 1. Observation

The toddler, especially if a 'terrible 2' year old, is unlikely to cooperate fully. Balance, gait, dexterity and speech can often be assessed by indirect observation while taking a history. The examiner may ask for your observations.

## 2. Engaging the child

Start with the parent. The child is more likely to be approachable if a friendly rapport is established between you and an adult he knows and trusts. Opening gambits such as 'How are you?' and 'How old are you?' or questions about travel, school, favourite TV programmes, pitched at an appropriate level, break the ice. Be friendly, smile! Toddlers often avoid direct eye gaze, or get upset if you look directly at them, so go along with them until they get used to you.

## 3. Touching

Not infrequently, small children resent or even fear a stranger touching them. Start with the hands. A game like 'round and round the garden', or for the feet 'this little pig went to market', works well.

## 4. Examining

Be gentle, doing 'easy' bits to begin with. Ears and throat or a rectal examination come last. Be an opportunist: do not expect to be allowed to do things in order.

Undressing can be upsetting, so ask the parent, if one is present, to undress the child. Removing a single garment at a time usually maintains cooperation.

Palpating the abdomen or listening to heart sounds by coming round from behind the child, out of sight, may be successful in the fretting infant.

Demonstration of auscultation or looking at the ear on an adult, especially a parent, helps. Let the child play with your torch, sphygmomanometer bulb, stethescope, etc.

## 5. Height, weight and head circumference measurements
Always obtain these measurements and plot them on a centile chart.

Further hints on examination of specific organs and systems are given at the beginning of each section.

Good luck!

# Congenital abnormalities

## CAUSES OF CONGENITAL ABNORMALITIES

1. Unknown
2. Genetic
3. Chromosomal
4. Maternal
    (i) Drugs: thalidomide, norethisterone, antimetabolites
    (ii) Infection: cytomegalovirus, rubella, toxoplasmosis
    (iii) Metabolic: diabetes mellitus, phenylketonuria
    (iv) Exposure: radiation
5. Uterine
    (i) Moulding, e.g. talipes, dislocation of hips
    (ii) Amniotic bands, e.g. amputations, facial clefts

## INCIDENCE OF CONGENITAL MALFORMATIONS

Major malformations: 1 in 50 of all live births.
Minor malformations: 1 in 25 of all live births.
   Association of two or more major malformations occurs in 1 in 10;
therefore look carefully for abnormalities in other systems if one
organ/system is affected

## FETAL DEVELOPMENT AND MALFORMING (TERATOGENIC) AGENTS

Teratogenic agents related to stage of fetal development

| Age and stage of development | Teratogens and their effects |
| --- | --- |
| 0-3 weeks old, early embryo | Chromosomal abnormality or abortion likely from irradiation and antimetabolites |
| 4–9 weeks old, stage of organogenesis | Abortion<br>Major malformation, e.g:<br>   Thalidomide: phocomelia<br>   Alcohol: fetal alcohol syndrome<br>   Infection (toxoplasmosis, cytomegalovirus (CMV) and rubella): mental handicap, microcephaly, small for dates, deafness, cataracts (not in toxoplasmosis), and (in rubella) heart defects |
| 10–40 weeks fetal growth | Altered growth and organ injury, growth failure, e.g.:<br>   Stilboestrol: vaginal carcinoma<br>   CMV: encephalitis, pneumonia, hepatosplenomegaly |

## MODES OF INHERITANCE

### Autosomal dominant
Recurrence risk 1 in 2 if:
1. One parent has the disease, e.g. adult polycystic kidney, spherocytosis, Huntington's chorea
2. Neither parent affected, i.e. spontaneous mutation, is common, and the risk to the affected child's offspring is 1 in 2, e.g. achondroplastic child with normal parents
3. Grandparent and grandchild affected, 'skipped generation', i.e. parent appears normal or is slightly affected, e.g. von Recklinghausen's disease, or detected only by special investigation, e.g. a computed tomogram of the brain showing characteristic calcification in tuberous sclerosis

### Autosomal recessive
Recurrence risk 1 in 4.
   Each parent carries a single abnormal gene for a disease found only when present in a double dose. This is thus more likely in consanguinous unions
Examples: sickle cell disease, thalassaemia, cystic fibrosis, inborn errors of metabolism

**Sex linked**
Usually recessive, risk to boys 1 in 2. A condition carried on the X chromosome, which males show as they have only one in each cell. Female carriers appear relatively or completely normal unless only one X is present, as in Turner's syndrome (XO). Lyon's hypothesis is that only one X chromosome is 'active' in each cell, and the number of active abnormal Xs a carrier has determines whether she shows any signs of the disease.

Mother carrier:  1 in 2 boys affected
$X_h X$  1 in 2 girls carriers
Father affected:  all boys normal
$X_h Y$  all girls carriers

Examples: colour blindness, glucose 6-phosphate dehydrogenase deficiency (p 63), X linked mental retardation (p 4), haemophilia, Duchenne's muscular dystrophy

**Multifactorial inheritance**
Interaction of an individual's genes with the environment. The likelihood of recurrence (risk) increases as the number of family members affected increases, at a rate peculiar to that condition
Example: spina bifida (vitamin/folic acid lack in genetically susceptible individuals?), recurrence risk for parents:
risk for the general population = < 1 per 1000
risk of another after 1 affected child born = 1 in 20
risk after 2 affected children born to them = 1 in 8

**'High' and 'Low' risk in genetic counselling**
For the purpose of counselling, geneticists suggest that a recurrence rate of more than 1 in 10 is a high risk, e.g. autosomal dominant, recessive and X linked disease. A low risk is less than 1 in 10, e.g. insulin dependent diabetes (about 1 in 10 to 1 in 20 in brothers, sisters and offspring of affected person).

The example of multifactorial inheritance, spina bifida, shows how a family's category of risk can change

## SOME SELECTED CHROMOSOMAL ABNORMALITIES

### 1. Down's syndrome
47 XY and sporadic in 95% with 1% recurrence, or translocation 46 XY in 3% and likely to recur in 10–100% because one parent carries the abnormal chromosome and has a 45 chromosome karyotype
Frequency: 1 in 600 live births, 1 in 50 in 40 year old mothers
Clinical: characteristic face, hands and feet. Hypotonia, mental retardation, congenital heart disease, duodenal atresia and Hirschsprung's disease

### 2.  Turner's syndrome (XO)
Frequency: 1 in 4000 live births, owing to loss of X or Y and unlikely to recur
   Neonate: low birth weight, low hair line, redundant skin folds, oedema of feet, coarctation of the aorta
   Childhood: *short stature, cubitus valgus, webbed neck,* occasional mental handicap. Ovarian dysgenesis causes failure of pubertal development

### 3.  Klinefelter's syndrome (XXY)
Frequency: 1 in 2000 live births, recurrence unlikely
   Clinical: 'maleness' predominates because of the Y chromosome. Normal looking as boys, may be mentally slow, often tall. At puberty 'eunuch' like, with gynaecomastia, small infertile testes, rounded hips

### 4.  Familial fragile X syndrome in XY males (X linked mental retardation)
Frequency: 1 in 1000 males, X linked recessive, recurrence risk 1 in 2 for boys, carrier females may be mentally slow
   Clinical: educationally subnormal, large ears and heads, large testes in adults

### 5.  XYY syndrome
Frequency: 1 in 1000 males, recurrence unlikely
   Clinical: tall, otherwise normal looking. Behaviour often aggressive, occasionally 'psychopathic.'

# Newborn

**SOME NORMAL PHYSIOLOGICAL FINDINGS IN THE NEWBORN**

1. Urine
   Normally passed within 24 hours. Delay suggests renal tract outlet obstruction, renal dysgenesis, shock. Action: feel for distended bladder, do ultrasonography of kidneys.
   Kidney concentrating ability is up to 600 mosmol/kg water, twice the osmolality of plasma (300 mosmol/kg water). (Adult kidney can concentrate up to 1500 mosmol/kg water)
2. Meconium
   Within 24 hours about 95% of healthy term infants pass meconium. Delay suggests organic obstruction, meconium ileus (often due to cystic fibrosis), or Hirschsprung's disease. Action: plain $x$ ray examination of abdomen, consider surgical opinion, rectal biopsy and/or sweat test, but remember prematurity, asphyxia and opiates given to mother can cause delay
3. Weight
   Loss of 5–10% of body weight, regained by the 10th day of life is normal. Reduced intake, infection, and pyrexia, increased losses via urine, stool or skin may cause or contribute to excessive weight loss. Very low birth weight infants may lose up to 15% of body weight
4. Respirations
   30–50 per minute, mainly periodic
5. Heart rate
   120–160 beats per minute
6. Blood pressure
   75/50 mm Hg, lower in premature infants
7. Heart murmurs
   Heart murmurs, soft and vibratory systolic, are heard in most infants on the first day of life. Thus, murmurs may be of limited significance. Absence does not exclude serious heart anomaly where it would be expected, e.g. Down's syndrome. Similarly, in a cyanosed infant with signs of respiratory distress: when in doubt in the latter case a nitrogen washout or 'hyperoxia test' is indicated

Hyperoxia test: breathing pure oxygen for 20 minutes; a rise in arterial oxygen concentration is likely in respiratory disease, not with cardiac problems

8. Blood sugar
   term infant > 1.6 mmol/1
   premature > 1.1 mmol/1  } in the first 72 hours
   > 2.2 mmol/1 thereafter

## A SCHEME FOR EXAMINING THE NEWBORN — 'TOP TO TOE'

### Aim
To detect:
1. Congenital abnormalities, especially of limbs, hips, heart, abdomen and eyes
2. Transition to effective normal respiration
3. The effects of delivery and gestation on the infant
4. The presence of infection or disease

### Method
1. Progress from head to feet, turn over to look at the back, look for midline abnormalities, compare the 2 sides of the body
2. (i) Scrutinise the face and body for characteristics e.g. of Down's syndrome
   (ii) Colour:
      pallor  =  anaemia/shock/infection
      cyanosis  =  central/peripheral/traumatic (p 47)
      jaundice  =  visible if > 100 $\mu$mol/1 serum bilirubin. Normal in 15% of newborn infants. Age, maturity and severity determine action
      red  =  high packed cell volume e.g. small for dates, fetal transfusion, infant of diabetic mother

3. *Head*
   Measure occipitofrontal circumference with a paper or fibreglass tape, not cloth, tightly round maximum circumference = occiput to brow 1 cm above nasal bridge. Look for caput or cephalhaematoma. Feel anterior fontanelle for increased tension due to crying or raised intracranial pressure, or overriding of sutures from the birth, dehydration or brain not growing.
   (i) Face: birth marks, e.g. 'stork mark' normal, port wine stain abnormal; check each nostril for patency by occluding each nostril in turn with the mouth closed and seeing that the infant can draw breath. If in doubt pass a nasogastric tube.
   (ii) Eyes: slight discharge common; if profuse, persistent or purulent needs evaluation. Sit baby up to examine pupils for colobomata, eyes for glaucoma, and with the

ophthalmoscope on +10 lens at 10 cm elicit the red reflex
(the retinal reflection) and look for dark spots or absent reflex
due to presence of cataract(s)

(iii) Mouth: palate often has midline white 'dots', which are
epithelial cells and called Epstein's pearls; clefts start from
the uvula unless a hare lip is also present. Cleft palate may
accompany a small jaw in the Pierre Robin syndrome

(iv) Ears: low position in renal problems, simple shape in Down's
syndrome, note sinuses, accessory auricles, earhole patency

(v) Neck: look for sinuses, feel for sternomastoid 'tumour' in
lower third (though it is not usually felt in the first week),
swelling over clavicle due to its being fractured, and thyroid
enlargement-all abnormal (Fig. 15, p 56)

4. *Upper limbs*
   Symmetry, full extension, normal shape and number of digits

5. *Chest*
   (i) Observe colour, respiratory rate and effort and symmetry of
   chest movement.
   Asymmetry suggests pneumothorax, lung collapse or
   compression by a diaphragmatic hernia or lobar
   emphysema. Observation of abdominal movements is
   valuable as babies rely mainly on the diaphragm; a see-saw
   motion of chest 'down' — abdomen 'up' on inspiration
   indicates severe lung collapse, as in respiratory distress
   syndrome (RDS), or weak intercostal muscles. The anterior
   chest wall is mainly soft cartilage, accounting for the sternal
   indrawing seen in conditions like RDS.
   Auscultation: bronchial breath sounds are normal but
   fine crackles (crepitations) after the first few hours of life are
   not

   (ii) Pulse rate, volume, and presence of femoral pulses to
   exclude coarctation; detection of full peripheral pulses, e.g.
   dorsalis pedis in patent ductus arteriosus

   (iii) Heart examination (p 47). Ensure silence during
   auscultation, using nipple or teat if necessary

6. *Abdomen*
   This may be distended, and enlargement of liver (normally 2–3
   cm below the right costal margin) or asymmetry due to tumours
   often easily seen. Gently palpate in a stroking motion from
   below upwards to detect them.
   The kidneys can best be felt by a gentle pincer action (like
   squeezing a squash ball) between the thumb anteriorly and the
   fingers behind, supporting the back.
   Listen for bowel sounds

7. *Genitals*
Always check for ambiguity (p 36).
   In boys born at term the scrotum is large and hydrocoeles that resolve by a year are common.
   In girls a creamy white discharge from the vagina often becomes bloody after the first 2 days and resolves in 2–3 days due to oestrogen withdrawal; vaginal skin tags are common

8. *Anus*
Check patency and reflex tone

9. *Lower limbs*
Postural talipes is normal, but a foot that cannot move into the correct position on tickling, or spontaneously, and cannot be overcorrected by passive manipulation, requires an orthopaedic opinion.
   Check the number of digits

10. *Back*
Mongolian blue spot is normal; look for spinal deformity, spina bifida or overlying naevus/hairy patch; sacral dimple is common and is rarely a sinus, and therefore needs no action

11. *Neurology*
Findings are influenced by alertness, relation to last feed (sleepy if recent, irritable if due) and intercurrent illness.
   (i)  Behaviour
       a. Apathy        } from drugs, asphyxia, sepsis, metabolic
       b. Irritability  } upset, hungry, drug withdrawal, asphyxia/
       c. Jitteriness   } birth injury, sepsis, hypocalcaemia,
                          hypoglycaemia
   (ii) Movement
       a. Asymmetry, with lack of movement of one side of body
          = hemisyndrome due to asphyxia/birth injury
       b. Floppy frog posture (p 9, 25) in prematurity, acute illness,
          cerebral (brain) injury
       c. Hypertonic, extended arched body with fisting, in brain
          injury, drug withdrawal, fits, kernicterus
  (iii) Primitive reflexes
          Rooting reflex, sucking and swallow may be affected by
       prematurity, drugs, asphyxia, etc
          The Moro reflex: weakness or lack of abduction of the
       arms and legs and a failure of their return to a general
       flexed posture are useful in detecting neurological damage
       affecting movement in:
          one arm e.g. Erb's palsy of cervical nerves 5, 6

both arms e.g. bilateral Erb's palsy
arm and leg same side in hemiplegia
NB The Moro may disappear in cerebral injury
   Asymmetric tonic neck reflex (ATNR): should not be
obligatory, i.e. if baby cannot move out of an ATNR
spontaneously this is abnormal and due to raised
intracranial pressure, asphyxia or cerebral palsy
   Walking reflex: may be impaired by sciatic nerve or spinal
cord damage
   Tendon reflexes are normally brisk and symmetrical
(iv) Tone and power
   Pull baby to sitting position using the palmar grasp. The
arms, trunk and head flex forward. Lack of flexion or marked
head 'lag' is abnormal—except in an angry baby!
   Sitting up, the chin should rise off the chest and not snap
backwards in uncontrolled extension.
   Pick up the baby, prone, your hand under the abdomen.
The head and back should be in line horizontally, hips and
knees gently flexed.
   Causes of hypotonia and weakness include:
   a. Prematurity
   b. Drugs
   c. Acute illness, e.g. infection
   d. Asphyxia
   e. Neurological conditions, e.g. intraventricular
      haemorrhage (see floppy infants, p 25)
(v) Gestational age. Assessment is needed if deviation from
   mother's dates is suspected from the examination or baby's
   behaviour. The Dubowitz scoring system is the best known

12. *Hip examination* (Fig. 1)
   (i) Place the infant on a firm, flat surface, on his/her back.
      Ensure he/she is relaxed. Adduct and flex the hips and
      knees, then abduct them fully, looking for:
      (a) limitation of abduction in either hip (Fig. 1a)
      (b) a 'jerk' interrupting the smooth arc (Fig. 1b)
      (c) a 'clunk' as the head relocates
   (ii) 'Telescope' the flexed thigh, abducted 45 degrees, in
      towards the acetabulum, the pelvis held firmly with the
      other hand (Fig. 1b). Examine each hip separately
   (iii) Finally, again adduct the flexed hips and knees, and
      internally rotate the hips so that the dorsum of each foot
      faces the other. Thumbs on inner thighs, index and middle
      fingers on outer (lesser and greater trochanters
      respectively), press vertically downwards to dislocate the
      hips (Fig. 1c). Now abduct and externally rotate the thighs
      so the soles now face each other, meanwhile pressing

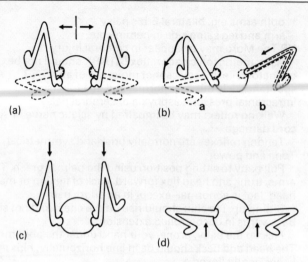

(a)    (b)  a    b

(c)    (d)

⟶ = DIRECTION FORCE IS APPLIED

**Fig. 1**

upwards with the fingers. As the hip returns a 'clunk' is felt (Fig. 1d).

Clicks arise from ligaments moving at hip and knee and are not generally thought significant

## DEFINITIONS AND MORTALITY RATES FOR 1983/4 IN ENGLAND AND WALES

Stillbirth: No signs of life immediately after expulsion from mother after the 28th week of gestation. Rate 6.0/1000 total live births and still births

Perinatal mortality: Number of stillbirths and deaths in the first week. Rate 11.0/1000 total live births and stillbirths

Neonatal mortality: Number of deaths in the first 28 days of life. Rate 6.0/1000 live births

Infant mortality: Number of deaths in the first year. Rate 10.0/1000 live births

## MAJOR CAUSES OF NEONATAL MORTALITY

1. Respiratory distress syndrome  } Prematurity
2. Immaturity
3. Asphyxia
4. Congenital abnormalities
5. Infection

## APGAR SCORE

| | No of points | | |
|---|---|---|---|
| | 0 | 1 | 2 |
| Appearance | White | Blue | Pink |
| Pulse | 0 | <100/minute | >100/minute |
| Grimace to clearing airways | 0 | Grimace | Cough, sneeze |
| Activity | 0 | Spontaneous flexion of limbs | Active |
| Respiratory effort | 0 | Irregular gasps | Regular, crying |

*Score*: assessed at 1 and 5 minutes

| | | | |
|---|---|---|---|
| 0–3 | at 1 minute | = | severe asphyxia |
| | at 5 minutes | = | risk of cerebral injury |
| | >10 minutes | = | cerebral injury and death likely |
| 4–6 at 1 minute | | = | mild to moderate asphyxia |
| 7–10 at 1 minute | | = | no significant asphyxia |

### Problems of the low birth weight infant

Of the 7% of all births weighing less than 2500 g, 60% are premature and 40% are small for dates

## PREMATURITY

### Definition
Less than 37 weeks' completed gestation

### Causes
1. Unknown
2. Uterus
    (i) Abnormal, e.g. cervical incompetence, double uterus
    (ii) Uterine distension, e.g. twins, polyhydramnios
    (iii) Premature rupture of membranes, includes (i)
3. Maternal
    (i) School age
    (ii) Previous premature delivery
    (iii) Closely spaced pregnancies
    (iv) Acute maternal illness, drug addiction
4. Fetal: congenital malformation, infection
5. Environmental: poverty
6. Therapeutic: rhesus isoimmunisation, diabetes, fetal distress

## Problems of the premature

*Early*
1. Immaturity
    (i) Respiration
        (a) Central control unstable (apnoea)
        (b) Surfactant deficiency (respiratory distress syndrome)
    (ii) Cardiovascular: bradycardias, hypotension, cardiac failure from patent ductus arteriosus from early fluid excess or reopens with hypoxia, anaemia
    (iii) Feeding: absent gag reflex before 34 weeks, functional ileus
    (iv) Liver: jaundice
2. Hypothermia: lack of brown fat and subcutaneous fat layer
3. Hypoglycaemia: lack of liver glycogen stores
4. Intraventricular haemorrhage: the less mature the more likely
5. Infection
6. Necrotising enterocolitis
7. Iatrogenic (see p 17)

*Later*
1. Bonding failure
2. Anaemia
    (a) Early dilutional = normochromic at 4−6 weeks
    (b) Late nutritional = hypochromic at 8−12 weeks
    (c) Haemolytic = folic acid deficient
3. 'Rickets of prematurity': probably inadequate phosphorus intake in very low birth weight infants.
    Classic rickets due to lack of vitamin D, more likely in premature infants because of rapid growth rate
4. Persistent patent ductus arteriosus: early fluid overload
5. Oxygen toxicity: retrolental fibroplasia, bronchopulmonary dysplasia (mechanical ventilation also implicated)
6. Brain damage: cerebral palsy, hydrocephalus from intraventricular haemorrhage

## SMALL FOR DATES

### Definition
Below the 10th centile for weight. These infants may be symmetrically small in all body proportions or light for dates, i.e. length and head circumference above the 10th centile

### Causes
1. Uterine
    (i) 'Placental insufficiency' = toxaemia, placental infarction, renal/essential hypertension
    (ii) Multiple pregnancy

2. Fetal
    (i) Congenital or chromosomal abnormality
   (ii) Infection by Toxoplasmosis, Others e.g. syphilis, rubella, Cytomegalovirus, *Herpes simplex* = TORCH
3. Maternal
   School age, poverty, smoking, race, high altitude, drugs, illness

**Problems of the small for dates**
1. Hypoxia
    (i) Intra uterine death during pregnancy or labour
   (ii) Polycythaemia
  (iii) Meconium aspiration causing pneumonia
2. Hypoglycaemia: inadequate glycogen stores, jittery, increased hunger drive
3. Hypothermia: lack of subcutaneous fat
4. Polycythaemia: results in jaundice, thromboses in the brain and heart failure
5. Congenital/chromosomal/infection problems: i.e. *examine very carefully!*

## BIRTH TRAUMA

1. Swellings, with usual time of identification
    (i) Caput: at birth, oedema of the scalp crossing suture lines
   (ii) Cephalohaematoma: 2–4 days old, subperiostial bleeding limited by suture lines
  (iii) Fractured clavicle: 1–20+ days, midclavicular swelling, from shoulder dystocia, breech extraction
  (iv) Sternomastoid tumour: 7–20+ days, lower third of the muscle. Intrauterine posture also a cause
   (v) Fat necrosis: 3–14 days, hard subcutaneous lump commonly over bone, skin overlying has a purplish hue
2. Common nerve palsies, usually identified at birth
    (i) Facial nerve, peripheral: asymmetrical crying face, open eye. (Absence of depressor anguli oris is associated with congenital heart disease, i.e. think of it if only mouth affected)
   (ii) Erb's palsy C5, 6–waiter's tip posture
  (iii) Klumpke's palsy C7, 8, T1–claw hand, flexed elbow, (plus Horner's syndrome = stellate ganglion involved)

## CAUSES OF FAILURE TO ESTABLISH RESPIRATION

1. Neurological
   a. Maternal medication/sedation
   b. Asphyxia/birth injury
   c. Prematurity

2. Respiratory
   a. Laryngeal spasm due to vigorous pharyngeal suction
   b. Pneumothorax
   c. Massive meconium aspiration
   d. Small lungs e.g. Potter's syndrome of absent kidney function, oligohydramnios, pulmonary hypoplasia and 'squashed baby'
   e. Diaphragmatic hernia
3. Circulatory: shock from blood loss; internal, into mother/twin
4. Metabolic
   a. Hypoglycaemia
   b. Acidosis

## CAUSES OF RESPIRATORY DISTRESS, APNOEA AND CYANOSIS

1. Respiratory
   (i) Parenchymal: RDS, meconium aspiration, pneumonia, pneumothorax
   (ii) Congenital structural: hypoplastic jaw and cleft palate (Robin syndrome), choanal atresia, oesophageal atresia, diaphragmatic hernia, Potter's syndrome
2. Cardiac
   (i) Cardiac failure
   (ii) Congenital heart disease
   (iii) Persistent fetal ciculation: full term moderately asphyxiated baby, normal heart and lungs, raised pulmonary vascular resistance
3. Neurological
   (i) Asphyxia/birth injury, CVA (intraventricular haemorrhage), drugs
   (ii) Seizure
4. Metabolic: hypoglycaemia, acidosis
5. Polycythaemia, anaemia (acyanotic)

## CAUSES OF APATHY, APNOEA, IRRITABILITY AND SEIZURE

1. Drugs and drug withdrawal
2. Asphyxia/birth injury
3. Infection
4. Metabolic: low glucose, sodium, calcium concentrations; acidosis; inborn errors
5. Intraventricular haemorrhage: premature, vitamin K deficiency
6. Congenital brain malformation, chromosome abnormality

## CAUSES OF JAUNDICE

Clinically recognised at 100 $\mu$mol/l serum bilirubin. 'Direct' or conjugated bilirubin should be less than 25 $\mu$mol/l

1. First day
   (i) Rhesus isoimmunisation, occasionally ABO incompatability
   (ii) Infection*, congenital (TORCH) and acquired
2. First week
   (i) Physiological
   (ii) Haemolytic: blood group incompatibility (* after exchange
        transfusions), red cell abnormality (e.g. glucose 6-phosphate
        dehydrogenase deficiency), spherocytosis (p 63)
   (iii) Extravasated blood reabsorption from bruises,
         cephalhaematoma, etc
   (iv) Infection*, congenital and acquired
3. Late onset after one week
   (i) Breast milk jaundice
   (ii) Infection*: urinary tract infection, herpes, hepatitis
   (iii) Hypothyroidism
   (iv) Biliary atresia*/neonatal hepatitis syndrome*

**Alternative strategy**
1. Prehepatic: haemolytic, extravisated blood, infection
2. Hepatic: physiological, congenital infection, hypothyroidism,
   neonatal hepatitis syndrome
3. Post hepatic: biliary atresia

## CAUSES OF ANAEMIA

**Definition**
At birth, a healthy mature infant's venous haemoglobin
concentration (Hb) is 19 g/dl while a premature infant's Hb is 16 g/dl.
Anaemia is less than 14 g/dl in first week

**Causes**
1. Haemorrhage
   (i) Into mother/twin
   (ii) Into baby: trauma, vitamin K deficiency, anticoagulants to
        mother
   (iii) Revealed: cord and placenta accidents, circumcision
2. Haemolysis
   (i) Infection
   (ii) Rhesus (direct Coombs' test positive), ABO etc
   (iii) Red cell defects: glucose 6-phosphate dehydrogenase
         deficiency, spherocytosis
3. Iatrogenic (blood taking)
4. Inadequate Hb production (rare)


(* = conditions in which 'direct' bilirubin concentration is raised)

## CAUSES OF HYPOGLYCAEMIA

### Definition
Diagnosed if true blood glucose in the first 72 hours is:

<1.5 mmol/l (30 mg/100 ml) over 2500 g  } clinical action if
<1.1 mmol/l (20 mg/100 ml) under 2500 g } <2.2 mmol/l
(40 mg/100 ml)

After 72 hours: <2.2 mmol/ l  (40 mg/100 ml)

### Causes
1. Delayed or inadequate feeds
2. Inadequate stores
    (i) Prematurity
    (ii) Small for dates
3. Increased requirement
    (i) Infection, RDS, hypothermia
    (ii) Infant of a diabetic mother

## CAUSES OF VOMITING

1. First 1–3 days
    (i) Feeding problem
    (ii) Gastric irritation, swallowed blood
    (iii) Obstruction: duodenal atresia (double bubble on x ray), meconium ileus, meconium plug, Hirschsprung's disease
    (iv) Functional ileus in the premature
    (v) Infection
    (vi) Neurological: asphyxia/birth injury, intraventricular haemorrhage
2. End of first week
    (i) Hiatus hernia
    (ii) Infection/necrotising enterocolitis
    (iii) Metabolic: renal failure, inborn errors of metabolism, e.g. congenital adrenal hyperplasia (p 37)
    (iv) Obstructive: Hirschsprung's disease

## CAUSES OF DELAY IN PASSING MECONIUM

1. Organic obstruction: anal stenosis or atresia
2. Meconium plug/meconium ileus – consider cystic fibrosis
3. Hirschsprung's disease

## CAUSES OF BLOOD IN STOOLS

1. Swallowed maternal blood
2. Infection/necrotising enterocolitis
3. Trauma, local e.g. hard stool, thermometer
4. Cow's milk allergy
5. Haemorrhagic disease of the newborn (vitamin K deficiency)
6. Acid ulceration: stress, hiatus hernia, Meckel's diverticulum

## CAUSES OF IATROGENIC DISEASE

### Historical
1.  Delayed feeding of premature infants: early hypoglycaemia, later increased incidence of cerebral palsy
2.  Deliberate hypothermia, incorrectly thought to reduce oxygen requirements; increased mortality
3.  Jaundice
    (i) Water soluble vitamin K causing haemolysis
    (ii) Drugs displacing bilirubin from albumin causing kernicterus, e.g. sulphonamides (but co-trimoxazole is still a potential hazard)
    (iii) Drug inhibition of glucuronidation by novobiocin

### Still topical
1.  Retrolental fibroplasia: oxygen toxicity plays a part
2.  Chloramphenicol excess: 'grey baby syndrome' = shock, due to cardiovascular collapse, fits
3.  Excessive separation of parents and infant

# Development and neurology

## NORMAL DEVELOPMENT

SOME MILESTONES IN NORMAL DEVELOPMENT.
Know at least one item per category for each age band

| Social | Hearing and speech | Vision and fine motor | Gross motor |
|---|---|---|---|
| **6 weeks** | | | |
| 1. Smiles (H) <br> 2. Coos (H) | 1. Stills to mother's voice or toy bell | 1. Follows face in 90° arc <br> 2. Stares intently | 1. Sat up: lifts head few seconds <br> 2. Examiner's hand lifting from under the body: head in line with trunk <br> 3. Primitive reflexes (p 8) present |
| **6 to 9 months** | | | 6 months: |
| 1. Objects go to mouth <br> 2. Enjoys bath and 'boo!' (H) <br> 3. No longer looks at hand; looks at foot <br> 4. Chews on biscuit (H) | 1. 6 months: 'ma,da' <br> 2. 9 months: babbles, 'Mama, dada', understands 'no-no', 'bye-bye' (H) <br> 3. Responds to own name <br> 4. Hearing test (p 22) | 1. Cover test (p 21) <br> 2. Eyes fix on pellet of paper <br> 3. At 6 months forgets falling object; by 9 months follows it <br> 4. 6 months: palmar grasp; 7 months: transfers; 9 months: index finger probing approach | 1. Rolls from back to front <br> 2. Sits alone few seconds <br> 3. Flexes head and trunk when pulled to sit <br> 9 months: <br> 1. Sits securely <br> 2. Pulls up on furniture to stand |

H = by history, objective enough for most cases; otherwise by direct observation

| Social | Hearing and speech | Vision and fine motor | Gross motor |
|---|---|---|---|
| **One year** | | | |
| 1. Comes when called | 1. Shakes head for 'no' | 1. Picks up crumbs with pincer grasp | 1. Pivots when sitting |
| 2. Lets go on request; finds hidden item | 2. Understands some words; says 1 to 3 words (H) | 2. Throws toys deliberately, watching fall to ground | 2. Walks alone or one hand held |
| 3. Dress; cooperates, pushing arm through sleeve | | 3. Holds 1 inch cube in each hand, bangs together, may make 2 cube high tower | |
| **18 months** | | | |
| 1. Cup: lifts, drinks and puts down (H) | 1. Jargons++ | 1. Fisted grasp of pencil, scribbles | 1. Walks well |
| 2. Spoon: feeds self (H) | 2. Points to 3 parts of body | 2. Points at wants | 2. Throws toy without falling |
| 3. Toilet: bowel clean, wet nappy discarded (H) | 3. Obeys single command 'get your cup', etc | 3. Picks up threads, pins, etc, neatly | 3. Climbs stairs (H) |
| 4. Copies: dusting, washing up, sweeping (H) | 4. Says 6 words; Echolalia | 4. Turns pages in picture book, 2 at a time | |
| | | 5. Tower of 3–4 x 1 inch cubes | |
| **2 to 2½ years** | | | |
| 1. Toilet: dry reliably by day, and tells in time (H) | 1. Many words | 1. Drawing: imitates vertical and horizontal line and circle | 1. Runs |
| 2. No sharing, plays alone, tantrums (H), demanding (H) | 2. Phrase of 2–3 words (H) | 2. Tower: 6–8 cubes | 2. Kicks ball |
| 3. Imaginative play | 3. Knows name | 3. Book: turns one page at a time | 3. Jumps on the spot |
| | 4. Understands 'give dolly a drink', i.e has inner language | | 4. Stairs: 2 feet per tread |
| | | | 5. Trike: pushes with feet |

| Social | Hearing and speech | Vision and fine motor | Gross motor |
|---|---|---|---|
| **3 to 3½ years** | | | |
| 1. Toilet: pulls pants down and up alone (H)<br>2. Eating: fork and spoon together (H)<br>3. Plays with other child, shares toy (H) | 1. Gives full name, sex<br>2. Counts by rote to 10<br>3. Uses 'me', 'I', 'you'<br>4. Understands on, under, back of, etc | 1. Colour matches 2+ colours correctly<br>2. Mature pencil grip; copies circle<br>3. Identifies square, triangle, although cannot draw them | 1. Stands on one leg momentarily<br>2. Stairs; adult style of ascent (H)<br>3. Trike: pedals (H) |
| **4 to 5 years** | | | |
| 1. Toilet: wipes own bottom (H)<br>2. Eating: knife and fork (H)<br>3. Dress: on and off unsupervised, except tie, laces (H)<br>4. Plays by the rules, competitive | 1. Gives name, address, age<br>2. Counts to 10<br>3. Grammar OK<br>4. Articulation almost mature | 1. Colours: matches 4+<br>2. Drawing: 4 years copies cross and square, by 5 years a triangle, draws a man with head, arms, legs and fingers | 1. Hops<br>2. Climbs trees (H)<br>3. Ball games, 'catch', etc (H) |

## VISION

### Vision testing
1. Corneal light reflex
   Reflection of ophthalmoscope light is in the same spot on each eye. Overcomes the common confusion caused by epicanthus, wide nasal bridge. Fig. 2a shows abnormal reflection
2. Cover test
   (i) Cover each eye in turn using a card, parent's hand or examiner's thumb swinging from one eye to the other with other fingers resting gently on crown of baby's head. Then
   (ii) Use a toy, keys or light to attract attention
   (iii) Hold the toy/keys at 30 cm
   (iv) Repeat at 2 m

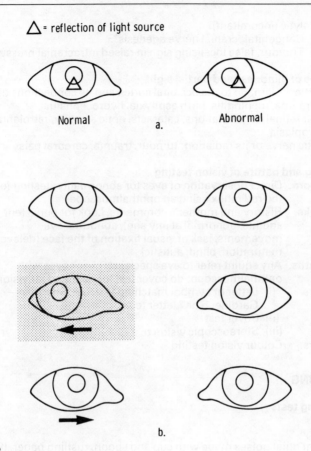

△ = reflection of light source

Normal                    Abnormal

a.

b.

**Fig. 2**

A latent squint is detected when the affected eye turns in or out, returning to its original position on being uncovered, as in Fig. 2b.

In manifest squint the cover test helps to identify alternating convergent squint, the eye affected in unilateral squint and vertical squint

NB: Resentment to covering 1 eye (the good one) may indicate abnormality in the other

**Causes of squint**
1. Non-paralytic (concomitant):
    (i) Failure of fusion of images (often inherited)
    (ii) Lens abnormalities (refractive errors, cataract)
    (iii) Nerve weakness due to febrile illness, head injury

2. Paralytic (incomitant):
   (i) Congenital: cranial nerve agenesis
   (ii) Tumour, false localising sign in raised intracranial pressure

**Causes of blindness and partial sight**
1. Cortical: damage to the occipital cortex and its connections due to trauma, meningitis, birth asphyxia, hydrocephalus
2. Eye: retinal degenerations, cataracts, optic atrophy, retrolental fibroplasia
3. Optic nerve or its radiation: tumour, trauma, cerebral palsy

**Timing and nature of vision testing**
**Newborn.**   Direct observation of eyes for abnormality; testing for the red reflex using an ophthalmoscope
**6 Weeks.**   History and mother's comments. Look for persistent squints (abnormal at any age), abnormal eye movements, lack of visual fixation of the face (delayed maturation, blind, autistic)
**6 Months.**   Any squint refer to eye specialist; check eyes with ophthalmoscope; do cover test for near and far vision
**4 Years.**       (i) Letter or symbol matching test, e.g. Sheridan—Gardiner 5 or 7 letter test
                       (ii) Cover test
                       (iii) Stereoscopic vision test
**8 Years.**   Colour vision testing


**HEARING**

**Hearing tests**

*Infancy*
Present quiet noises made with cup and spoon, rustling paper, high pitched rattle, whispered 's', 'oo' and baby's name. The head or eyes turn to the side tested
   7 months: at 50 cm from ear   } 45 degrees behind baby's ear and
   9 months: at 1 m from ear      } level with it

*Preschool (2½ to 3 years old)*
1. Identifying objects: points to common objects, the names of which have already been said, then repeated at quieter sound levels during the test
2. 'Go' and 'sss' games: conditioning the child to place an object (toy) in a box each time you say 'go' or 'sss' at successively quieter sound levels

### Causes of deafness/failed hearing test
1. Acute otitis media ⎫ conductive deafness
2. Serous otitis media ⎭
3. Congenital
   (i) Genetic, unknown – conductive and nerve deafness
   (ii) Infection, e.g. rubella, CMV – nerve deafness
4. Perinatal: asphyxia, hyperbilirubinaemia, drugs, prematurity –
   nerve deafness

## DEVELOPMENTAL WARNING SIGNS
1. Family history, e.g. deafness, cataracts
2. Mother worried
3. Motor problems
   (i) Persistence of reflexes (Moro, automatic walking, palmar
       grasp, tonic neck reflexes in cerebral palsy (CP)) after time for
       disappearance
   (ii) Early hand preference before 1 year old in hemiplegia
   (iii) Not sitting unsupported by 9 months or walking by 18
        months in CP, mental retardation, floppy baby (p 25)
   (iv) Boy not walking by 18 months: consider Duchenne's
        muscular dystrophy and test blood creatine phosphokinase
        activity (CPK)
4. Hearing and speech problems: see delayed speech (p 25)
   (i) No tuneful, double syllable babble ('mmumum, dadad') by
       10 months
   (ii) Less than 6 words at 18 months
   (iii) No 2–3 word sentences by 2½ years
5. Visual difficulties (see p 22)
6. Social unresponsiveness: causes include deprivation, mental
   retardation, failure to thrive (p 34), autism

## CAUSES OF DELAYED DEVELOPMENT
By and large prematurity should be taken into account when
assessing developmental progress, i.e. a 3 month premature infant
at 6 months old will be at least a 3 month level of ability, usually
more
1. Idiopathic: constitutional, familial (affecting *one* field, e.g. bottom
   shuffler, catching up later)
2. Deprivation
3. Mental retardation
4. Specific abnormality, e.g. blind, deaf, cerebral palsy

## CAUSES OF DETERIORATION IN DEVELOPMENT

1. Emotional shock, deprivation
2. Failure to thrive
3. Neurological: epilepsy, status epilepticus, drugs, any severe insult, e.g. trauma, meningitis
4. Metabolic: inborn errors, e.g. phenylketonuria, lead poisoning
5. Endocrine: hypothyroidism in infancy

## CAUSES OF PLAGIOCEPHALY ( squint skull)

1. Intrauterine moulding
2. Lying mainly on the one side: hypotonia, cerebral palsy
3. Sternomastoid shortening ('tumour')
4. Craniostenosis — premature fusion of one skull suture

## CAUSES OF A SMALL HEAD

1. Normal development: constitutional, familial, small body
2. Abnormal development likely: microcephaly
   (i) Familial and sporadic
   (ii) Brain injured: trauma, asphyxia, infection, etc
   (iii) Mental retardation syndrome, e.g. Down's

## CAUSES OF A LARGE HEAD

1. Normal development: constitutional, familial (measure circumference of parents' heads)
2. Failure to thrive
3. Abnormal development likely
   (i) Hydrocephalus
   (ii) Subdural collections
   (iii) Tumour

## CAUSES OF DELAYED CLOSURE OF THE ANTERIOR FONTANELLE

(Normally achieved by 18–24 months)
1. Rickets
2. Hypothyroidism
3. Hydrocephalus

## CAUSES OF MENTAL HANDICAP

1. Prenatal
   (i) Genetic:
      a. chromosomal, e.g. Down's syndrome, X linked mental retardation (p 4)
      b. familial, e.g. tuberous sclerosis, inborn errors of metabolism

   (ii)  Congenital infection: TORCH (p 13)
   (iii)  Alcohol, drugs, e.g. phenytoin
2.  Perinatal: asphyxia, birth injury, prematurity
3.  Postnatal: meningitis, head injury, seizures, lead

## CAUSES OF SLOW SPEECH DEVELOPMENT

1.  Deprivation, emotional
2.  Developmental delay, often familial
3.  Deaf, usually secretory otitis, others (p 23)

## CAUSES OF FLOPPY INFANTS

1.  Non-neurological: failure to thrive, acute infection
2.  Brain abnormality: injury, mental retardation, Down's syndrome, cerebral palsy
3.  Spinal: trauma, polio, spinal muscular atrophy
4.  Peripheral nerve: polyneuritis
5.  Neuromuscular junction: myasthenia gravis
6.  Muscular dystrophies

## CAUSES OF SEIZURES BY AGE

### Stage of brain maturation related to seizure type

| | |
|---|---|
| Neonatal (age up to 4 weeks) | Asphyxia/birth injury, infection, hypoglycaemia, hypocalcaemia, intracranial haemorrhage, drug withdrawal |
| Infantile spasms (age 3–9 months) | Idiopathic in ⅓ cases, tuberous sclerosis, brain malformations/injury, congenital infection, encephalopathy |
| Febrile convulsion (age 1–5 years) | Fever usually due to infection, and not in the central nervous system |
| Petit mal (age 3–15 years) | Idiopathic |
| Benign focal epilepsy of childhood (age 7–10 years) | Idiopathic |

Photosensitive    Idiopathic, but may be found in other forms of
epilepsy          epilepsy and especially brain damage
(age 8–14 years)

### Seizures largely independent of age
Grand mal         Genetic in many

Temporal lobe     Idiopathic, genetic or symptomatic of some
epilepsy          underlying cause

## CAUSES OF BACTERIAL MENINGITIS BY AGE

0–3 months
{ Gram negative; *Escherichia coli*, proteus,
  pseudomonas
  Gram positive; group B streptococcus
  *Haemophilus influenzae*
  Neisseria *meningitidis* }

Older ages        *Streptococcus pneumoniae*
                  *Mycobacteriam* tuberculosis (rare but important)

## CAUSES OF HEADACHE

1. Tension, especially likely in school refusal (p 28)
2. Migraine
3. Raised intracranial pressure: tumour, abscess
4. Post-traumatic
5. Infection: meningitis
6. Sinusitis, dental caries
7. Hypertension (rare)
8. Intracranial bleed (rare)

# Behaviour

**CAUSES OF ENURESIS**

1. Physiological delay (with family history usual)
2. Pyschological stress
3. Organic
   (i) Urinary tract infection
   (ii) Mental retardation
   (iii) Neurological, e.g. spina bifida, epilepsy
   (iv) Structural lesion, e.g. posterior urethral valves
   (v) Diabetes mellitus

**CAUSES OF FAECAL SOILING**

1. Untrained
2. Organic: anal fissure resulting in constipation and overflow incontinence, Hirschsprung's disease
3. Psychological
   (i) Retention — may lead to fissure
   (ii) Antisocial

**CAUSES OF RECURRENT ABDOMINAL PAIN/PERIODIC SYNDROME**

1. Psychological stress
   (i) Home: marital discord, separation experiences, family illness, poor parent–child relationship
   (ii) School: bullying, problems in discipline and learning
   (iii) Sexual abuse
2. Migraine tendency: personal and family history
3. Constipation or *abnormal* bowel action
4. Medical causes of acute abdominal pain (p 58)

## CAUSES OF SCHOOL REFUSAL

1. School refusal: separation anxiety, refuses to leave
2. Truancy (leaves home and fails to arrive or absconds later): educational difficulties, psychosocial problems common
3. Educational difficulties, e.g. slow, chronic illness, poor vision, unsuspected hearing loss, emotional stress, dyslexia, etc, poor teaching, large class

# Growth and nutrition

## NORMAL GROWTH

Infant weight gain: 30g/day (1 oz) from 10th day
  By 5 months: birth weight × 2
  By 1 year: birth weight × 3

## NORMAL REQUIREMENTS

Calculate according to *expected* weight for gestational age
1. 150–200 ml/kg/day for first 6 months
2. 110 kcal (460 kJ)/kg/day for first year; thereafter 1000 kcal (4200
   kJ) + 100 kcal (420 kJ) for each year of life, e.g: @ 2 years = 1000
   + 200 kcal/day; @ 11 years = 1000 + 1100 kcal/day.
   (Approved powdered formula milks made up to manufacturers
   instructions contain 110 kcal/150 ml, similar in calories to mature
   breast milk)
3. Weaning: first solids introduced from 3–6 months, breast
   feeding gradually reduced from 6–12 months old
4. Doorstep (unmodified) cow's milk can be introduced from 6
   months old
5. Vitamins
   British DHSS vitamin drops – 5 drops daily, from 1 month to 2
   years – contain:
     A = 700 IU
     C = 20 mg
     D = 400 IU
   Recommend for infants drinking doorstep milk, Asians and
   breast fed infants of poorly nourished mothers.
   Very low birth weight premature infants have additional needs
   for folic acid and vitamin E for the first 2–3 months
6. No added sugar or salt in solids
7. Iron: for premature infants and twins in the first 6–12 months
8. Fluoride: as one part per million tap water, or if necessary, as
   drops. Now ubiquitous in toothpaste

## HAZARDS OF COW'S/FORMULA MILK

1. Psychologically may be less satisfying than breast feeding
2. Infection
    (i) During preparation
    (ii) Lack of anti-infective properties
3. Obesity
4. Cow's milk protein allergy
5. Anaemia
    (i) Iron deficiency (but formula milks now fortified with iron)
    (ii) Cow's milk protein allergy
6. Hypocalcaemia
7. Hypernatraemia


## BENEFITS OF BREAST FEEDING

1. Nutritionally balanced
2. Anti-infective properties: macrophages, lactoferrin, secretory
    IgA, lysosyme lactobacilli
        (May be especially valuable for premature infants in prevention
        of infection and necrotising enterocolitis)
3. Psychological
4. Anti-allergic
    NB: Remember the hazards: early vitamin K deficiency,
    underfeeding, maternal medication excreted in breast milk


## NUTRITIONAL DISORDERS

### Vitamin A
A rare deficiency except in the developing world, still a major cause
of blindness in some countries
Clinical: Night blindness, photophobia, dry corneas
    (xerophthalmia), keratomalacia; slow development; horny skin,
    respiratory infections

### Scurvy
Lack of vitamin C results in bleeding gums, purpura from capillary
bleeds, pseudo-paresis due to subperiosteal bleeds.
    Exceedingly rare in developed countries. Prevention: see p 29
Treatment: 0.5 g vitamin C a day

### Rickets
1. Due to vitamin D deficiency
At risk: Asian infants and adolescents, from inadequate intake, lack
    of sun, phytates in the diet; premature infants; less commonly,
    those taking anticonvulsants, malabsorbing (coeliac, etc)
2. Vitamin D resistant rickets, renal rickets (chronic renal failure,
    renal tubular acidosis) – all rare

3. Substrate deficiency. Very low birth weight premature infants may be phosphate deficient

Clinical: Frontal bossing, anterior fontanelle slow to close, enlarged wrists, swelling of rib ends ('rickety rosary'), symmetrical bow legs, hypotonic muscles

Cause: In nutritional rickets low vitamin D intake causes inadequate calcium absorption from the gut; parathormone rises to mobilise calcium from bone and causes renal excretion of phosphate

Serum biochemistry shows:
a. Calcium normal, phosphate low
b. Alkaline phosphatase raised (upper limit in premature infants up to 5 times adult maximum, children twice that of adults, and again rising much higher in puberty)
c. Vitamin D low

Radiology shows:
a. Loss of normal bone density
b. 'Cupped' appearance at end of long bones due to widening of metaphysis
c. Irregular calcification of the epiphyseal plate
d. Greenstick fractures

Prevention: see p 29

Treatment: 1500 IU vitamin D a day

**Anaemia**

Iron lack in premature infants, twins, delayed weaning (see p 29).
Pale, increased respiratory rate, palpable spleen, systolic murmur.

**Marasmus**

Lack of protein and *calories*

Causes:
1. Placental, in utero (see small for dates–p 12)
2. Postinfective diarrhoea
3. Chronic infection e.g. UTI, TB, malaria
4. Malabsorption (e.g. cystic fibrosis)
5. Neglect

Clinical: Hungry unhappy infant, no oedema; length and weight below 3rd centile, i.e. stunted due to prolonged starvation; more acute weight loss results in 'baggy' skin folds

Treatment: Feed to *expected* weight, high calorie and protein formula, avoid hypothermia, investigate for associated infection/deficiency of iron, vitamins and possible cause. In developing country education may prevent this

**Kwashiorkor**

Lack of protein greater than calories, i.e. at weaning in developing countries, 1–3 years old. Black skin depigments irregularly, hair reddens, generalised oedema, large liver, prone to infection, which often precipitates kwashiorkor

**Obesity**
Causes
1. Overeating
2. Constitutional, familial and racial
3. Emotional, compensatory overeating
4. Endocrine, e.g. Cushing's syndrome – iatrogenic from steroids.
   Beware the short fat child!

# GROWTH

**Measurement**
A single measurement of height and weight allows a static
comparison with the rest of the population using a standard growth
chart.
   Repeated measurements allow assessment of the rate of growth
or growth velocity. The minimum interval between such
measurements is 3 months using a stadiometer
*Parental height comparison* will show whether the child is on the
expected mid-parental centile, which can be roughly calculated from
the standard chart as follows:
Boys  (i)   plot mother's height on the right hand margin
      (ii)  add 12.5 cm to this, make a mark
      (iii) plot father's height, make a mark
      (iv)  expected height centile is mid point between the two
            marks
Girls (i)   plot father's height and deduct 12.5 cm, mark
      (ii)  expected height centile is mid-way between the mark and
            mother's height

*BONE AGE* is the expected 'average' skeletal maturity at a given
chronological age, both expressed in 'years'. Use in assessing cause
of abnormal growth pattern:
1. Normal bone age, i.e. same as chronological age in short stature
   of family or genetic cause
2. Delayed bone age proportional to actual height, i.e. the height
   plotted on the chart at that bone age is within expected centiles
   (Fig. 3)
3. Delayed bone age, the actual height progressively falling away
   from expected velocity in failure to thrive (p 34), hypothyroidism,
   growth hormone deficiency (Fig. 4). Without treatment final adult
   height may be reduced
4. Advanced bone age in virilisation and precocious puberty (p 35)
*CATCH-UP growth* occurs for a finite period after suppression by
subnutrition or severe illness and is an increased growth velocity
towards expected stature

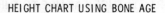

HEIGHT CHART USING BONE AGE

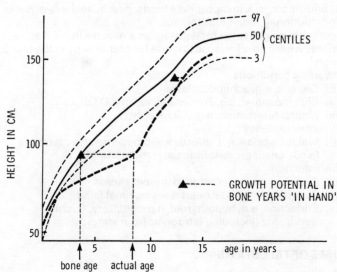

**Fig. 3**

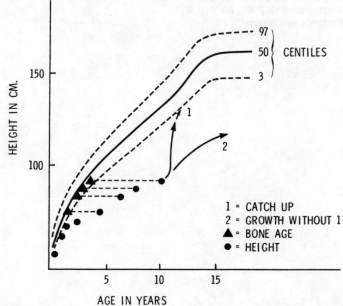

**Fig. 4**

## CAUSES OF SHORT STATURE/FAILURE TO THRIVE

1. Subnutrition: lack/inappropriate foods, psychosocial deprivation
2. Constitutional: individual, familial
3. Low birth weight/small for dates (or as a mistake in premature infants where no allowance is made for prematurity in the first 2 years)
4. Dwarfing conditions
   (i) Genetic, e.g. achondroplasia
   (ii) Chromosomal, e.g. Turner's syndrome (XO)
   (iii) Mental retardation, e.g. microcephaly
5. Systemic diseases
   (i) Malabsorption, e.g. infective and postinfective diarrhoea (p 59), coeliac, cystic fibrosis, Hirschsprung's
   (ii) Infection
   (iii) Asthma – poorly controlled/steroid excess
   (iv) Cyanotic congenital heart disease, renal failure
   (v) Endocrine, e.g. hypothyroid, hypopituitary, Cushing's Syndrome (including iatrogenic from steroids)

## CAUSES OF TALL STATURE

1. Constitutional: individual, familial
2. Endocrine, e.g. precocious puberty (at first) (p 35), thyrotoxicosis, congenital adrenal hyperplasia (p 37)
3. Chromosomal: XXY, XYY (p 4)
4. Marfan's syndrome

# Sexual differentiation and puberty

## SOME NORMAL PUBERTAL EVENTS

### Girls
1. Onset from 8-14 years with breast, genital, then pubic hair the usual order of development
2. Maximum growth achieved before menarche, only 6 cm on average after onset of menses
3. Menarche mean age is 13 years. The bone age at which menarche occurs corresponds to that at 13 years old

### Boys
1. The first sign of puberty is usually testicular enlargement at 10-14 years with an increase in volume to 4 ml (about a medium sized or stuffed olive). Accurate estimation is obtained with an orchidometer, a string of ovoids of increasing volume 1-24 ml, used for comparison by palpation
2. Gynaecomastia is common and normal and may be unilateral
3. The sex difference in height is largely due to 2 extra years' prepubertal growth because boys start puberty 2 years later, on average

## PRECOCIOUS PUBERTY

Present if pubertal changes occur before 8 years in girls, 10 years in boys; commoner in girls. Pathological cause more likely in boys (60%) than girls (20%)

NB: Early breast development (premature thelarche) from 1–2 years old and axillary or public hair *alone* (adrenarche) from 7 years old is usually normal

### Causes of precocious puberty
1. True (mediated through gonadotrophins)
    (i) Physiological: constitutional, familial, obesity
    (ii) Hypothalamic: injury, hydrocephalus, postinfective, tumour
    (iii) Tumour producing gonadotrophins

2. False, or pseudo (sex hormones present in excess independent of hypothalamic or gonadotrophin control). Boys' testes remain small unless 1 has a tumour, girls may be virilised
    (i)   Adrenal, e.g. congenital adrenal hyperplasia (p 37)
    (ii)  Gonadal tumours of testes or ovaries
    (iii) Drug: anabolic steroids

## DELAYED PUBERTY

Absence of any signs by 14 years old, or prolonged arrest of progress after the initiation of puberty

### Causes of delayed puberty
1. Physiological: constitutional or familial
2. Chronic disorders, e.g. malnutrition, coeliac, Crohn's disease, diabetes mellitus, anorexia nervosa
3. Hypothalamic/pituitary lack of gonadotrophins
4. Gonads unable to produce sex hormones despite adequate gonadotrophins, e.g. streak ovaries in Turner's syndrome
5. End organs unresponsive, e.g. testicular feminisation

## VAGINAL DISCHARGE

Clear or white discharge in small amounts is physiological, and may cause a stain on the pants

### Causes
1. Physiological
2. Non-specific vaginitis
3. Infection: gonococcal, streptococcal, monilia, herpes, threadworm
4. Foreign body

## CAUSES OF AMBIGUOUS GENITALIA
1. Virilisation of girls: congenital adrenal hyperplasia (p 37)
2. Feminisation of boys
    (i)   undescended testes: normal, anorchia, XXY
    (ii)  testicular feminisation: an X linked disorder of end organ unresponsiveness to testosterone in an XY person – short blind-ended vagina, no uterus, little pubic hair, testis may be found in inguinal hernia
    (iii) errors in testosterone synthesis
3. Hermaphrodite, i.e. mixed gonads often with mosaic sex chromosomes

# Endocrinology

## AGE OF ONSET OF ENDOCRINE PROBLEMS

### Neonatal – infancy

1.  Infant of diabetic mother
    Longer and heavier than expected, early hypoglycaemia, respiratory distress syndrome and jaundice more likely, higher incidence of congenital anomalies, e.g. sacral agenesis (absent sacrum)
2.  Hypothyroidism
    Goitre – mother taking antithyroid drugs, familial disorders of thyroid synthesis; prolonged neonatal jaundice in a large baby likely
    Later in infancy: constipated, hypotonic, growling slow cry, pale (anaemia), coarse skin and hair, cold, large tongue, umbilical hernia, delayed bone age and general development slow, poor growth, thyroid stimulating hormone (TSH) level raised on Guthrie test, low thyroxine (T4)
3.  Congenital adrenal hyperplasia (CAH)
    21-hydroxylase deficiency commonest, inherited in autosomal recessive mode, results in low cortisol, high androgen (male sex hormone) production, causing
    (i)   Virilisation of girls, and deeply pigmented genitals in boys at birth
    (ii)  Shock from salt loss, with vomiting, dehydration, poor weight gain and lethargy from end of first week of life
    (iii) Sudden unexpected death
    Later: accelerated growth and pseudo-precocious puberty (p 36). Final adult height shorter if untreated
    Biochemistry: raised serum potassium, urea; lowered sodium, bicarbonate; occasionally hypoglycaemia.
    Very high serum 17-hydroxyprogesterone best test for 21-hydroxylase deficiency in the neonate

**Preschool (1–4 years)**
Growth hormone deficiency, ideopathic
   Commoner in boys, fall off in growth from begining of second
year, often insidious. Short, fat, large looking head, small genitals,
well. May not be recognised until school age. Growth velocity <5 cm
a year. Bone age not always delayed

**School age**
1. Diabetes mellitus, insulin dependent
   Few days or weeks of poor appetite, weight loss, polydipsia,
   onset enuresis, monilial vulvitis, short history of vomiting,
   abdominal pain, deep sighing breathing, coma
      Investigation and treatment: see p 99
2. Hypothyroidism
      Causes: failing, small thyroid; autoimmune disease; lack of
   iodine (see goitre).
      Growth retarded with 'infantile' proportions (long trunk, short
   legs); bone age (p 32) retarded; excessively well behaved, no
   retardation in intellect; pale, constipated, dry skin, etc;
   occasionally precocious puberty
3. Hyperthyroidism
   Diffusely enlarged thyroid; accelerated growth, advanced bone
   age; in addition to usual signs in adults, affecting the eyes and
   metabolism, early symptoms include disturbed behaviour,
   deterioration in handwriting and schooling
4. Cushing's syndrome
      Cause: commonly caused by iatrogenic steroid administration,
   e.g. for asthma, Still's disease.
      Growth failure, osteoporosis; immunosuppression, increased
   danger from infection; adrenal suppression; moon face, buffalo
   hump, obese trunk, hirsute, acne; thin limbs from muscle
   wasting, weak, personality change; hypertension; red face (high
   Hb), striae

## CAUSES OF GOITRE

1. Euthyroid
      (i) Physiological at puberty
      (ii) Autoimmune thyroiditis (later hypothyroid)
2. Hypothyroid
      (i) Iodine deficiency
      (ii) Antithyroid drugs
      (iii) Enzyme deficiency, usually familial
3. Hyperthyroid: thyrotoxicosis

## CAUSES OF HYPOGLYCAEMIA

Neonatal: p 16
Older ages: p 75

# Respiratory disease

## EXAMINATION

### Nose
Shape, deviation and nasal discharge (unilateral, mucopurulent/ bloody in foreign body or choanal atresia). A transverse crease suggests allergy from frequent rubbing of the nose with the flat of the hand (allergic salute).

The mucosa can be seen with the auriscope light, and in older children the speculum used to assess it: pink is normal, red is infected, pale and swollen is allergic/ vasomotor rhinitis; and Little's area often has scars or ulcers from nose picking and associated bleeds.

Polyps occur in older children with cystic fibrosis. Mouth breathing in mid-childhood suggests adenoidal hypertrophy. Tonsils and adenoids largest at 6–8 years

### Ears
Shape, position (below a line level with the outer canthus of the eye suggests renal abnormality) and size noted.

To examine the tympanic membrane in the younger child demonstrate examination on a doll/parent and invite imitation, then you and the child jointly handling the auriscope or you alone examine the child's ear.

If potentially uncooperative the infant or child is held sat facing forwards or sideways on an adult lap, head against the adult chest with one hand, the other hand round the child's hands and trunk.

To straighten the external auditory canal for the best view: infant - pull the ear lobe downwards; child - pull pinna (top) up and back.

To prevent injury or pain from a sudden movement of the child rest the knuckles of the hand holding the auriscope on the cheek or scalp

*Causes of changes in appearance of the tympanic membrane (TM)*
Grey drum, with cone of light reflex, is normal
1. Pink injection around the edge of the TM in crying infant
2. Red uniformly in acute otitis media
3. Dark, almost black in impending perforation or blood behind TM

4. Black hole is a perforation
5. Dull grey retracted TM by blocked eustachian tube
6. Dull grey bulging TM, often bubbles or a fluid level in secretory otitis

**The chest**

Respiratory rate:
| | |
|---|---|
| infancy | 40 ± 10 per minute |
| child | 30 ± 10 per minute |
| adult | 15 ± 5 per minute |

*1. Observation*

Rounded diameter in infancy, oval thereafter.

Costochondral junctions seen or palpated along a line from mid-clavicle obliquely down to the anterior axillary line at the bottom of the rib cage. The junctions are enlarged in rickets (rickety rosary). Harrison's sulci are the depressions along the lower rib cage at the insertion of diaphragmatic muscle, normal or due to chronic respiratory or cardiac disease, or rickets.

As the front of the chest is of soft cartilage the sternum is indrawn in generalised lung collapse (e.g. respiratory distress syndrome) or airways obstruction (e.g. epiglottitis); hyperinflation in bronchiolitis or asthma produces a pigeon chest appearance

*2. Percussion*

Infants: chest wall and contents hyper-resonant, increased if lying on a mattress, which acts as a sounding board, and percussion not very helpful. Can identify the upper border of the liver on the right (6th space anteriorly, decreasing dullness up to the 4th space)

Children: findings in pneumonia, effusions, and hyperinflation similar to adults

*3. Auscultation*

Breath sounds are bronchial in infancy, and remain so over the mid-clavicular areas in small children. Similar sound heard in consolidation, lobar collapse.

Upper respiratory noises may be referred and often cause confusion but are coarse crackles, not medium or fine crackles due to bronchitis/bronchopneumonia.

Fine crackles are heard in pneumonia, and expiratory wheeze with fine crackles in infants with bronchiolitis

## COMMON CAUSES OF RESPIRATORY DISEASE

Relationship of respiratory disease to age and common causes

| Disease | Age | Causal agents |
|---|---|---|
| 1. Recurrent otitis media, upper respiratory tract infections | All ages | Streptococcus pneumoniae, H. influenzae, respiratory syncitial virus (RSV), Adenovirus, influenza. parainfluenza |
| 2. Epiglottitis | 3–7 years | H. influenzae |
| 3. Laryngotracheo bronchitis | 1–3 years | RSV, parainfluenza, influenza, rhinoviruses |
| 4. Bronchiolitis | Infant | RSV |
| 5. Asthma | > 1 year | Viruses; exercise/cold air; allergies; emotion |
| 6. Pneumonia | Neonate | E. coli, pseudomonas species, Group B haemolytic streptococcus |
| | Infant | RSV, Influenza, Staphylococcus aureus, S. pneumoniae |
| | Child | RSV, Influenza, Parainfluenza, S. pneumoniae, Mycoplasma pneumoniae |

## CAUSES OF ACUTE COUGH

1. Acute upper and lower respiratory tract infection
2. Asthma
3. Foreign body

## CAUSES OF CHRONIC COUGH

1. *Postnasal* drip: infected or atopic adenoids and sinuses
2. Asthma
3. Persistent infections: pertussis syndrome, *M. pneumoniae*, tuberculosis (TB), psittacosis
4. Foreign body
5. Cystic fibrosis
6. Aspiration syndromes: hiatus hernia
7. Habit

## DIFFERENTIATION OF THE MAJOR CAUSES OF ACUTE STRIDOR

Epiglottitis (E), laryngotracheobronchitis (LTB) and foreign body (FB) above the carina

|  | E | LTB | FB |
|---|---|---|---|
| Age | 0–3 years | 3–7 years | $\geq$ 6 months |
| Onset | In hours | 1–2 days | Sudden, may be missed |
| Respirations | Laboured | Increased | Variable |
| Cough | + | ++ | +++ |
| Drooling | +++ | − | − |
| Appearance | Pale, toxic | Normal/anxious | Normal |
| Voice | Hoarse, weak | Hoarse | May be aphonic |
| Hypoxia | Frequent | Unusual | Variable |
| X ray  Neck | Large epiglottis | Normal | Radio-opaque FB? |
| X ray  Chest | Normal | Inflammatory changes in half the children | Lung or lobe overinflated/ collapsed if FB moves below carina |

## CAUSES OF ACUTE STRIDOR

1. Acute laryngotracheobronchitis
2. Acute epiglottitis
3. Foreign body
4. Rare but important: diphtheria, retropharyngeal abscess, acute angioneurotic oedema

## CAUSES OF CHRONIC STRIDOR

1. Weak cartilage in the wall: laryngomalacia
2. Internal narrowing
   (i) Subglottic stenosis or haemangioma
   (ii) Vocal cord paralysis: recurrent laryngeal nerve damage, raised intracranial pressure
   (iii) Laryngeal web, papilloma
3. Compression from surrounding structures: vascular ring, tumour

## CAUSES OF RECURRENT WHEEZE

1. Asthma-wheezy bronchitis-bronchiolitis
2. Aspiration, e.g. hiatus hernia
3. Foreign body
4. Cystic fibrosis
5. Compression from mediastinal masses, glands

## CAUSES OF LYMPHADENOPATHY

1. Normal to have small glands in the various sites
2. Infection
3. Eczema
4. Malignancy
5. Drugs, serum sickness
6. Systemic juvenile chronic arthritis — Still's disease (p 52)

## X RAY APPEARANCES OF NOTE

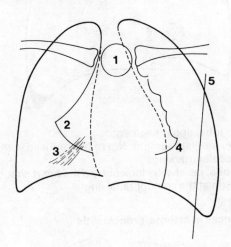

**Fig. 5**

## Common normal X ray appearances

1. Ossification centre, upper sternum. Coin-like, it may be confusing if the child is slightly rotated and it is then seen in the lung field
2. Sail sign of a normal thymus
3. Slightly increased bronchovascular markings in the right lower zone *only*, no thickening or segmental opacities in health
4. Wave sign of normal thymus indented by overlying intercostal muscles
5. Fat line extends beyond lung fields, and lung markings extend to the periphery unlike in pneumothorax

## X ray signs of pneumonia in sites often overlooked

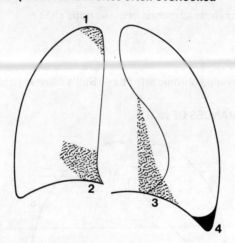

Fig. 6

1. Right upper lobe, upper segment
2. Middle lobe, medial segment. Not to be confused with normal bronchovascular markings
3. Left lower lobe, i.e. always look *behind* the heart shadow
4. Small effusion at the costophrenic angle

## X ray appearances in asthma/bronchiolitis

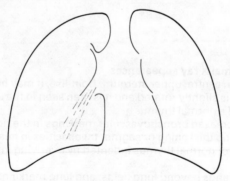

Fig. 7

Features to identify:
    barrel chest shape
    horizontal ribs
    flat diaphragms
    prominent hilar bronchovascular markings
    hypertranslucent lung fields

## Common causes of asymmetric lung field translucency on X ray

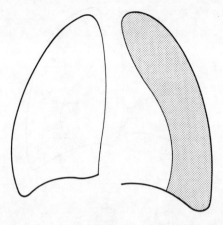

**Fig. 8**

1. Compensatory hyperinflation for collapse of other lung
2. Pneumothorax
3. Ball-valve effect:
   (i) Foreign body
   (ii) Hilar glands compressing bronchus
   (iii) Congenital lobar emphysema

1. Pneumonia
2. Tension pneumothorax *other* lung, this one collapsed
3. Aspiration into lung, with its collapse
4. Effusion, similar to aspiration but more uniform opacity and horizontal fluid level with upward curve at lung edge

## X ray appearances in cystic fibrosis

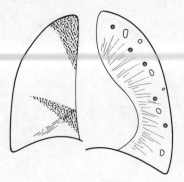

Fig. 9

*Early signs*: hyperinflation; segmental/lobar collapse; especially right upper and middle lobes

*Later signs*: cystic areas, thickened bronchial walls, well seen end on. Left upper and right middle particularly affected. Scars show as thickened lines radiating from the hilum

## X ray appearances in staphylococcal pneumonia

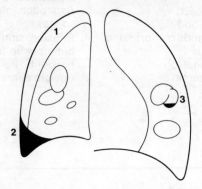

Fig. 10

1. Pneumothorax
2. Effusion (empyema)
3. Cysts, often fluid filled
   NB: (1) plus (2) = pyopneumothorax

# Cardiology

## NORMAL VALUES

| Age (years) | Heart rate (beats per minute) | Blood pressure (mm Hg) |
|---|---|---|
| 0–2 | 120–100 | 80/50–90/60 |
| 3–5 | 100 | 90/60 |
| > 5 | 90–80 | 90/60–110/80 |

## EXAMINATION

1. Cyanosis = > 5 g/dl of desaturated haemoglobin (Hb) in the newborn with a high haematocrit, otherwise > 1.5 g/dl with normal haemoglobin concentration as long as child is not anaemic
   - (i) Central: tongue is the most reliable site for confirmation
   - (ii) Peripheral cyanosis: normal in healthy neonates
   - (iii) Traumatic cyanosis: cord compression makes head and neck blue and purpuric
   - (iv) Differential cyanosis: pink head and neck, blue below a coarctation of the aorta with patent ductus arteriosus (PDA)
2. Pulse
   Always check femoral pulses. Absence, weakness or delay compared with right radial or axilla pulse suggests coarctation. Check blood pressure (BP) (see below); lower BP in legs confirms coarctation
3. Blood pressure (BP)
   Cuff size two thirds the length of the outer aspect of the upper arm or thigh, ensuring its bladder encircles the limb. BP in legs normally a few mm Hg higher than arms
   Procedure in infants: Auscultation often difficult in babies, so flush Bp may be used. Raise the limb, apply cuff, inflate, lower the limb - a red blush as the cuff is slowly deflated approximates to the mean systolic BP. Doppler is now replacing this time honoured method.

Procedure in children: Toddlers and children respond well to making a game of it. 'Let's play the silver line game. You look for it [the mercury column], and I'll listen.' Inflate, check radial or dorsalis pedis pulse as you deflate to get idea of systolic (may be the only reading!). Palpate for brachial or popliteal pulsation, apply stethoscope to the spot and repeat. Diastolic may be indeterminate in otherwise healthy children, i.e. does not disappear until down to 20–30 mm Hg

4. Apex
   4th or 5th interspace, within the nipple line. Always check for dextrocardia
5. Liver edge
   Easily palpated in infants and toddlers (p 55), 1–3 cm below the right costal margin in the nipple line
6. Jugular venous pressure
   Useful in older children. Hepatomegaly is a more reliable sign of congestive cardiac failure in the 0–2 year old
7. Oedema
   Infants and sick children lie horizontally, so look for pitting oedema over sacrum, or swelling around eyes
8. Surgical scars tell their own story
   (i)   Cut down sites for drips, femoral scars for catheters
   (ii)  Sterniotomy scar from cardiac surgery
   (iii) Thoracotomy scar for PDA, to make shunts for cyanotic congenital heart problems, lung or mediastinal problems
   (iv)  Neck and upper abdomen scars for lines and CSF shunts

## AUSCULTATION

1. Serious heart disease *Does* occur without a murmur. Myocarditis is then more likely than congenital lesion
2. Rapid heart rate may obscure abnormal heart sounds and murmurs
3. Venous hums are often continuous and subclavicular. If heard on the left may be confused with a PDA. Turning the head or lying down alters a hum but not a ductus murmur
4. Innocent murmurs
   (i)   Asymptomatic
   (ii)  No thrill
   (iii) Localised to the left sternal border and apex
   (iv)  Short and musical, mid-systolic and grade ⅜ or less
   (v)   Varies with sitting up and lying down, often disappears on lying
5. Third heart sound is physiological, in early diastole, at the apex

## IMPORTANT PATHOLOGICAL FINDINGS

1. First sound
   An ejection click follows immediately after it in poststenotic dilatation of the pulmonary artery or aorta

2. Second sound
   a. Loud in pulmonary hypertension
   b. Soft and apparently single in pulmonary stenosis
   c. Fixed split on breathing in/out in atrial septal defect
3. Murmurs

Ejection systolic: increased flow or stenosis of pulmonary or
aortic valve

Pansystolic: (i) shunt from higher to lower pressure, e.g.
ventricular septal defect (VSD), atrial septal
defect primum (ASD), patent ductus arteriosus
(PDA)
(ii) regurgitant,
e.g. mitral incompetence

Diastolic, early: regurgitant aorta or pulmonary valve
middle: increased flow from shunts (VSD, ASD, PDA)
late: obstructed flow across tricuspid or mitral
valve

## CONGENITAL HEART DISEASE

Acyanotic, shunts and obstructive lesions
cyanotic lesions

Acyanotic congenital heart disease – shunts*

|  | Age specific symptoms | Clinical signs of note |
|---|---|---|
| Patent ductus arteriosus | Premature infants: Recurrent apnoea, persistent RDS, congestive cardiac failure (CCF) Infant: 'Chesty', failure to thrive (FTT). CCF Adult: Breathless, cyanosis, subacute bacterial endocarditis (SBE) | Pulses: bounding. Thrill: 'to and fro' left infraclavicular area, same as: Murmurs: pansystolic, becoming continuous and 'machinery' like ± mid-diastolic flow murmur from mitral valve at apex |
| Ventricular septal defect | 3 months: Large VSD, reduced pulmonary vascular resistance causes acute CCF ± cyanosis Infant: Moderate VSD, 'chesty', FTT, CCF Child: Small VSD, asymptomatic, risk of SBE | Pulse: normal, or weak and rapid. Apex: thrusting, laterally displaced. Thrill: lower left sternal edge. Heart sounds: 2nd is widely split, from increased filling of right ventricle. Murmurs: harsh pansystolic ± mid-diastolic mitral flow at apex |

*NB: Chest x ray in all but the mildest cases show varying degrees of cardiac enlargement, pulmonary plethora and prominent pulmonary vessels

## Acyanotic congenital heart disease — shunts (contd.)

|  | Age specific symptoms | Clinical signs of note |
|---|---|---|
| Ostium secundum and atrial septal defect | Child: asymptomatic Adult: Breathless from pulmonary hypertension | Pulse: normal, no thrill. Heart sound: wide fixed split of 2nd sound from conduction delay (right bundle branch block). Murmurs: mid-systolic at 2nd left interspace, ± mid-diastolic tricuspid flow at lower right sternal edge |
| Ostium primum | Infant: 'Chesty', FTT, CCF Child: Progressive cyanosis as shunt reverses from the pulmonary hypertension | As for secundum +, if mitral valve is cleft (common). Thrill: left sternal edge. Murmur: apical pansystolic from mitral valve incompetence |

## Acyanotic congenital heart disease – obstructive

|  | Age specific symptoms | Clinical signs of note |
|---|---|---|
| Aortic stenosis (various causes) | Infancy: (i) Valvular: CCF if a severe stenosis (ii) Supravalvular: asymptomatic, unusual face, retarded development, ↑ Ca + + (William's syndrome) Child/adult: Valve/obstructive Cardiomyopathy: dizzy, angina, sudden death | Pulse: small volume. 'plateau' Apex: thrust. Thrill: left sternal edge radiating up to the neck Heart sounds: soft 2nd aortic part, the usual split may be reversed (i.e. ↑ on expiration) Murmur: ejection systolic radiating to the neck |
| Coarctation of the aorta | Infancy: Breathless, CCF (VSD often present) Child/adult: Asymptomatic, ruptured berry aneurysm, SBE | Differential cyanosis in neonates, i.e. pink above the ductus and blue below Pulse: absent/weak/delayed femorals, raised BP in upper limbs Hyperdynamic neck pulsations Apex: thrusting. Murmur: ejection systolic radiates through to the back |
| Pulmonary stenosis | Infancy: If severe, acute CCF, ± cyanosis due to right to left shunt via foramen ovale; otherwise asymptomatic in children Adult: CCF, arrhythmias | Jugular venous pulse: large 'a' wave Right ventricular heave Thrill: 2nd left interspace Heart sounds: second sound normal aortic part absent or soft pulmonary part Murmur: ejection click, then systolic ejection in 2nd interspace |

Acyanotic congenital heart disease — obstructive (contd.)

|  | Age specific symptoms | Clinical signs of note |
|---|---|---|
| Hypoplastic left heart | Few days old (2–6): CCF pale, severe acidosis like sepsis or an inborn error | Shock, low BP, death in days |

Cyanotic congenital heart disease

|  | Age specific symptoms | Clinical signs of note |
|---|---|---|
| Transposition of the great arteries | Cyanosis from birth or shortly after, proportional to shunt through foramen ovale, ductus arteriosus or a VSD. Breathless, CCF | Cyanosis, clubbing. 100% oxygen: cyanosis not improved, may even worsen cyanosis by closing the ductus (i.e. ductus dependant). Heart sounds: single. Murmur: often absent. Chest x ray: 'egg on side' shaped heart |
| Fallot's tetralogy (pulmonary infundibular stenosis, VSD, right ventricle hypertrophies, aorta overrides) | Infant: Progressively deeper cyanosis, weeks or few months old. Cyanotic 'spells' from infundibular spasm. Childhood: 'Squatting' after exertion, SBE, cerebral abscesses, polycythaemia | Cyanosis, clubbing. Right ventricular heave. Heart sound: single 2nd. Murmur: ejection systolic at 3rd, left interspace. Chest x ray: 'boot shaped' heart |
| Eisenmenger syndrome of irreversable pulmonary hypertension | Infant or child with VSD, transposition of the great arteries, PDA, common atrioventricular canal in Down's syndrome. Torrential flow of blood through lungs causes the pulmonary vessels to thicken, irreversibly. Cyanosis, CCF follow | Right parasternal (ventricular) heave and the pulmonary valve closing can be palpated. Heart sound: loud pulmonary 2nd. Murmur: ejection systolic ± early diastolic from pulmonary regurgitation |

## CAUSES OF CARDIAC FAILURE

1. Stress: fever, hypoxia, infection, acidosis
2. Anaemia
3. Fluid overload
4. Cardiac
   - (i) Neonatal: PDA, hypoplastic left heart, coarctation
   - (ii) Infancy: VSD, myocarditis
   - (iii) Child: systemic hypertension, pulmonary hypertension, bacterial endocarditis

## CAUSES OF CYANOSIS

1. CNS depression: drugs, trauma, asphyxia
2. Seizures
3. Respiratory disease
4. Stress: infection, hypoglycaemia, adrenal crises
5. Polycythaemia in the newborn
6. Cardiac
   (i) Neonatal: transposition of the great arteries (TGA), persistent fetal circulation
   (ii) Infancy: Fallot's tetralogy
   (iii) Child: pulmonary hypertension

## CAUSES OF RAISED BLOOD PRESSURE

### Acute
1. Renal: acute glomerulonephritis, trauma
2. Burns
3. CNS: infection, space occupation
4. Haemolytic uraemic syndrome (p 72)

### Chronic
1. Renal: infected, scarred, obstructed and congenitally abnormal kidneys, tumours
2. Vascular: renal artery stenosis, coarctation of the aorta
3. Corticosteroids (including Cushing's syndrome)

## CLINICAL CHARACTERISTICS OF SYSTEMIC JUVENILE CHRONIC ARTHRITIS (STILL'S DISEASE), RHEUMATIC FEVER AND HENOCH-SCHONLEIN (ANAPHYLACTOID) PURPURA

|  | Still's | Rheumatic fever | Henoch-Schonlein |
|---|---|---|---|
| Cause | Autoimmune | BHS | BHS, viral, allergy |
| Age | 1–5 years | 4–7 years | >1 year, peak at 5 years |
| Fever | Diurnal/any pattern | Sustained | Normal/raised |
| Rash | Maculopapular | Erythema marginatum | Urticarial/purpuric |
| Joints | Neck, knee, hip, foot, hand | Wrist, elbow knee, ankle | Wrist, ankle, knee |
| RES | Glands, hepato-splenomegaly | Liver ++ if in heart failure | No enlargement |
| Heart | Pericarditis | Pericarditis and carditis | No involvement |

| | Still's | Rheumatic fever | Henoch-Schonlein |
|---|---|---|---|
| Urine | Normal | Normal | Haematuria |
| Abdomen | Occasional pain | Normal | Acute pain common |
| Duration | Months | Days<weeks | Days>weeks |

BHS = B haemolytic streptococcus
RES = Reticulo-endothelial system


## REVISED JONES' CRITERIA FOR DIAGNOSIS OF RHEUMATIC FEVER

### Major criteria
1. Arthritis
2. Carditis
3. Erythema marginatum
4. Subcutaneous nodules
5. Sydenham's chorea

### Minor criteria
1. Previous history of rheumatic fever
2. Arthralgia
3. Increased erythrocyte sedimentation rate (ESR)
4. Prolonged PR interval on electrocardiogram (ECG)
5. Fever

### Evidence of streptococcal infection
1. Positive culture
2. Scarlet fever rash
3. Elevated *Antistreptolysin O* antibodies (ASOT)

For diagnosis: 2 major criteria; or 1 major + 2 minor criteria + evidence of preceding streptococcal infection

# Gastroenterology

## EXAMINATION

### 1. Mouth

Ask the child to show the teeth first, then to say 'ah' or 'eh'.
Demonstration by a parent or attendant helps. Crying may reveal
all! Alternatively, have the child held sat facing forward on
parent's lap, one arm encircling the child's arms and upper trunk,
the other hand restraining the forehead against the adult's chest.
This hold also enables the *ears* to be inspected by rotating the
head from side to side (p 39).

The buccal mucosa is inspected for Koplick's spots, thrush, torn
frenulum from trauma, etc

### 2. Teeth

By the age of 2 years all 20 milk teeth should be present; eruption
of the permanent teeth occurs from 6–13 years, excluding third
molars

### 3. Gums

Asian and African children often have dark brown–blue
pigmentation, with bluish pink interdental papillae, but the
underside and edges of the tongue should be pink. At the gum
margin a black line is seen in lead poisoning, but is also a normal
finding in African children

### 4. Abdomen

(i) *Inspection*

A thin abdominal wall with intestinal 'ladder' pattern is
common in premature infants and some term infants. The
rectus muscles are often 1–2 cm apart (divarication of the
recti) in infancy. Umbilical hernias reduce easily, rarely
obstruct and generally resolve by 2 years – or 5 years in
Africans, who also tend to have a pot bellied appearance due
to a physiological lumbar lordosis

*(ii) Palpation*
The liver (hatched area) is a large abdominal organ crossing the midline. Place the right hand gently on the abdomen from the child's right side, and using the radial side of the index finger to feel for the liver edge, advance from the groin, hand parallel to the right costal margin. Percuss along the same line of advance to confirm size. Normal values are 3 cm below the costal margin in the nipple line in infancy, 2 cm at 1 year and 1 cm at 5 years.

The spleen is palpable in normal infants, though seldom more than 1 cm, and occasionally in health after 1 year old, although it frequently enlarges during infections (p 61). It is smooth in outline at first, becoming notched in later childhood.

The kidneys are lower in infants than children, are easily palpated and fetal lobulation may be felt. In the neonate, flex the thighs with one hand and with the other palpate the kidneys with the thumb in a gentle pincer action against the fingers of that hand, which slip under the back to support it. The right kidney is lower than the left, and both move headwards on expiration.

The bladder is often palpable in early childhood as it is an intra-abdominal organ. Ensure it disappears on voiding, especially in boys, to help exclude outlet obstruction

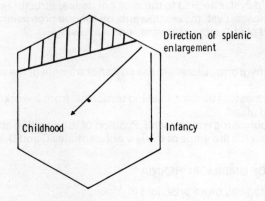

**Fig. 11**

## CAUSES OF COMMONER SWELLINGS IN THE NECK

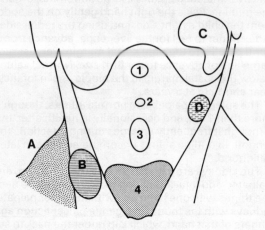

**Fig. 12**

**Midline**
1. Submandibular lymph gland
2. Dermoid cyst, attached to the skin, not deeper structures like 3
3. Thyroglossal cyst, moves upwards on tongue protrusion
4. Thyroid gland, moves upwards on swallowing

**Lateral**
A. Cystic hygroma, usually in the posterior triangle of the neck from birth
B. Sternomastoid tumour, causing torticollis, from 2 weeks old
C. Parotid gland
D. Jugulodigastric lymph gland. Position of the swelling above (C) or below (D) the angle of the jaw differentiates C and D

## CAUSES OF UMBILICAL HERNIA
1. Physiological, more prevalent in Africans
2. Prematurity
3. Down's syndrome
4. Hypothyroidism
5. Mucopolysaccharidoses (gargoylism)

## CAUSES OF INGUINAL SWELLINGS

1. Enlarged lymph glands
2. Inguinal hernia
3. Hydrocoele (causes confusion, and inguinal hernia may be associated with it)
4. Undescended testis

## CAUSES OF HAEMATEMESIS

NB: Exclude colouring from drinks or food
1. Swallowed blood
    (i) Neonate: maternal at birth or cracked nipple
    (ii) Epistaxis
2. Vomiting repeatedly, acute gastritis
3. Ulceration
    (i) Hiatus hernia
    (ii) Drugs: aspirin, iron poisoning
    (iii) Peptic ulcer
4. Munchausen by proxy (factitious bleeding)
5. Rare but important: oesophageal varices, bleeding disorders (p 64)

## CLINICAL FEATURES OF HIATUS HERNIA VERSUS PYLORIC STENOSIS

NB: Feeding mismanagement and urinary infections share many of these symptoms and signs

|  | Hiatus hernia | Pyloric stenosis |
| --- | --- | --- |
| Age at onset | First week | 2–6 weeks |
| Sex | Males = Females | Firstborn males (M:F = 5:1) |
| Family history | – | In 20% |
| Vomiting | Continuous, wells up, fresh/altered blood if ulceration present<br>No bile | Forceful, soon after feeds. Altered blood occasionally<br>No bile |
| Nutrition | Slowly progressive failure to thrive, repeated aspiration and pneumonia occur | Acute weight loss, dehydration, metabolic alkalosis |
| Stools | Occasionally constipated, altered blood | Starvation stools |

## ABDOMINAL EXAMINATION IN PYLORIC STENOSIS

**Inspection:** visible peristalsis, moving transversely from the left upper quadrant downwards towards the midline above the umbilicus

**Palpation:** from the baby's left hand side place the palm of your left hand on the abdomen with fingers curling round the lateral edge of the right rectus muscle midway between the lower edge of the rib cage and the level of the umbilicus. The pylorus muscle is towards the back, contracts into a rubbery pea shape then relaxes ('have I lost it?'), only to harden up again, every few minutes

## CAUSES OF VOMITING

1. Non-organic
    (i) Infants: overfeeding, posseting, rumination
    (ii) Children: self induced, overeating
    (iii) Adolescents: anorexia/bulimia nervosa
2. Infection: gastroenteritis or as parenteral response to urine infection, otitis media, etc
3. Gastrointestinal disorders
    (i) Medical: hiatus hernia, food allergies (cow's milk protein intolerance), coeliac disease
    (ii) Surgical: pyloric stenosis, acute obstruction, appendicitis; repeated episodes may occur in malrotation
4. Cough: pertussis, asthma
5. Migraine, cyclical vomiting
6. Medication
7. Uncommon but important
    (i) Metabolic: diabetes mellitus, uraemia, congenital adrenal hyperplasia
    (ii) Raised intracranial pressure

## COMMON CAUSES OF ACUTE ABDOMINAL PAIN

1. Medical (exclude coughing)
    (i) Infection: gastroenteritis, 'mesenteric adenitis', lower lobe pneumonia, urinary tract infection, acute hepatitis
    (ii) Constipation
    (iii) Henoch-Schonlein (anaphylactoid) purpura
    (iv) Acute nephritis
    (v) Rare but important: e.g. diabetes mellitus, sickle cell crisis, lead poisoning
2. Surgical
    (i) Acute appendicitis
    (ii) Obstruction: intussusception, strangulated inguinal hernia, volvulus
    (iii) Renal: hydronephrosis, colic
    (iv) Torsion of testis or ovary

## CLINICAL FEATURES OF APPENDICITIS VERSUS MESENTERIC ADENITIS

|  | Appendicitis | Mesenteric adenitis |
|---|---|---|
| Recurrent | – | Previous episodes common |
| Upper respiratory tract infection | Maybe | Within 24 hours, cervical glands + |
| Temperature and appearance | Usually 38°C; in preschool up to 40°C; ill, becomes toxic | 39–40°C common, flushed |
| Vomiting | Frequent | Unusual |
| Abdominal tenderness, guarding | Marked, usually very distressed, localised to right side, young child pushes hand away + + | Vague, generalised, periumbilical, often comes and goes |
| Rectal examination | Localised tenderness on right | No localised tenderness |

## CAUSES OF RECURRENT ABDOMINAL PAIN (p 27)

## CAUSES OF ACUTE DIARRHOEA

1. Starvation stools (mucousy, watery and green)
2. Infection: rota and enterovirus, *E.coli*, shigella, salmonella, campylobacter, giardia, amoeba
3. Food poisoning toxins: staphylococcal
4. Parenteral response to infection, e.g. pneumonia, otitis media, etc
5. Surgical: pelvic appendicitis, intussusception, Hirschsprung's disease

## CAUSES OF CHRONIC DIARRHOEA

1. Failure to gain or actual loss of weight and persistent loose watery stools for more than 2 weeks
   (i) Enteric infections: see above; note that immune deficiency may be present
   (ii) Postenteric infection: lactose and cow's milk protein intolerance, transient gluten enteropathy
   (iii) Inflammatory bowel disease: food allergies, ulcerative colitis, Crohn's disease,
   (iv) Malabsorption: coeliac disease, cystic fibrosis
2. Normal growth, loose or semiformed stools
   (i) Chronic non-specific toddler's diarrhoea
   (ii) Constipation with overflow
   (iii) Laxative abuse, a form of Munchausen by proxy

## CONFIRMATION OF CARBOHYDRATE MALABSORPTION
### (e.g. post enteritis)

Collect a sample of fluid stool by reversing a plastic disposable nappy. Mix 1 part stool with 2 parts tap water in a test tube and add a Clinitest Reagent tablet. More than 0.5% is a positive result

## CHARACTERISTICS OF CYSTIC FIBROSIS AND COELIAC DISEASE

|  | *Cystic fibrosis* | *Coeliac (untreated)* |
|---|---|---|
| **Newborn** | Meconium ileus | – |
| **Infant** | Failure to thrive from birth; recurrent pneumonia | Failure to thrive from introduction of gluten, usually at 3–4 months old |
| 1. Stools | Often abnormal from birth, diarrhoeal, very smelly, oily like melted butter | Normal until gluten introduced; become pale and bulky; not oily |
| 2. Appetite | Voracious | Poor |
| 3. Chest | 'Bronchitis' frequent, i.e. recurrent bronchopneumonia | Normal |
| 4. Social | Lively | Withdrawn, 'difficult' |
| 5. Others | Rectal prolapse, salty taste to skin, heat exhaustion | Anaemia, rickets, long eyelashes |
| **Child,** above plus: | | |
| 1. Height | Relatively preserved | Short |
| 2. Puberty | Delayed, males sterile | Delayed, amenorrhoea common in females |
| 3. Abdomen | Meconium ileus equivalent; biliary cirrhosis and portal hypertension cause enlarged spleen and oesophageal varices | Distended, liver edge often impalpable. Buttock wasted |
| 4. Others | Cor pulmonale; nasal polyps; diabetes mellitus | School failure from lethargy |
| Screening | Neonatal blood trypsin level raised (Guthrie card may be used) | 1 hour after oral D-xylose, blood level <20 mg/100 ml (not 100% reliable) |
| Diagnosis | Sweat sodium 70 mmol (mEq)/l or more on at least 100 mg of sweat | Villous atrophy, heals on diet, relapses on gluten, i.e. 3 jejunal biopsies |

## CAUSES OF RECTAL BLEEDING OR BLOOD IN THE STOOL

NB:  (i)  Exclude coloured drinks, beetroot
     (ii) Fresh bleeding is usually large bowel, malaena may be
          from a more proximal site higher up
1. Local: constipation, anal fissure
2. Swallowed blood from epistaxis
3. Dysentery
4. Acid ulceration: hiatus hernia, peptic ulcer, Meckel's
   diverticulum, aspirin
5. Intussusception

## COMMON CAUSES OF ENLARGED LIVER AND/OR SPLEEN

1. Infection: hepatitis A and B, infectious mononucleosis, malaria,
   septicaemia
2. Haematological: mainly spleen in spherocytosis, sickle cell,
   severe iron deficiency anaemia, thrombocytopenia
3. Congestive cardiac failure, mainly liver
4. Malignancy: leukaemia, lymphoma, secondary deposits in the
   liver, e.g. neuroblastoma

## CAUSES OF JAUNDICE IN INFANTS AND CHILDREN (neonates p 14)

### Unconjugated ('indirect' reading hyperbilirubinaemia)
1. Haemolytic: spherocytosis, sickle cell, thalassaemia, glucose
   6-phosphatase deficiency
2. Metabolic: Gilbert's disease (dominantly inherited diminished
   ability of uptake of bilirubin by liver cells)

### Conjugated ('direct') bilirubin > 25 $\mu$mol/1 (1.5 mg/100 ml)
1. Infection: hepatitis A and B, urinary infection, malaria
2. Drugs
3. Metabolic: alpha 1-antitrypsin deficiency (hepatitis like syndrome
   in infant, emphysema in adult) and other inborn errors, inherited
   in autosomal recessive manner
4. Biliary obstruction: biliary atresia
5. Chronic inflammatory disease, e.g. chronic active hepatitis

# Haematology

## NORMAL CHANGES IN HAEMATOLOGY

Birth:       Haemoglobin (Hb) 19 g/dl at term, 16 g/dl in premature
             infants.
             Lymphocytes predominate from the end of the first
             week of life through to late childhood.
             HbF (fetal haemoglobin) more than 50% of total Hb
1st year:    Hb falls to its lowest level at about 2 months, and
             thereafter averages 11 g/dl. HbF is 5% of total at 6
             months
Childhood:   12 g/dl

## CAUSES OF ANAEMIA

1. Decreased production, especially iron deficiency anaemia
2. Increased destruction (haemolysis)
3. Blood loss

## CAUSES OF HYPOCHROMIC (IRON DEFICIENCY) ANAEMIA

1. Nutritional
   (i)  Prolonged milk feeding and foods containing inadequate
        iron
   (ii) Malnutrition
2. Prematurity
   Inadequate stores = 'late anaemia' at 8–12 weeks. ('Early
   anaemia' at 4–6 weeks is dilutional owing to rapid growth and
   therefore normochromic)
3. Chronic infection, e.g. urinary tract infection (more often presents
   as *normochromic* anaemia)
4. Malabsorption, e.g. coeliac disease
5. Cow's milk protein intolerance
6. Peptic ulceration, e.g. hiatus hernia, Meckel's diverticulum
   causing loss of iron via bleeding

## CAUSES OF HAEMOLYTIC ANAEMIA, BY AGE AT PRESENTATION

### Neonatal
1. Acquired
   (i) Immune: rhesus, ABO
   (ii) Infection, congenital (TORCH p 13), and acquired
2. Genetic
   (i) Enzyme deficiency, e.g. glucose 6-phosphate dehydrogenase deficiency (G6-PD) - sex linked, Mediterranean, Asian and black populations mainly affected. Haemolysis is spontaneous in newborn, later episodes precipitated by drugs, fava beans and sepsis
   (ii) Spherocytosis - autosomal dominant, large spleen, jaundice and anaemia, gall stones in adults

### Infancy
   (i) Infection, acute, e.g. septicaemia, malaria. Meningococcaemia may cause disseminated intravascular coagulation
   (ii) Genetic: sickle cell disease and thalassaemia both become manifest from 6 months as HbF production falls
   (iii) Haemolytic uraemic syndrome (p 72)

### Childhood
1. Acquired
   (i) Infection, acute: see 2 (i) above
   (ii) Autoimmune Coombs positive anaemia after infections, e.g. mycoplasma, viral, also idiopathic, or may be drug induced
   (iii) Drugs, e.g. penicillin, sulpha, nitrofurantoin
2. Genetic, e.g. sickle cell, thalassaemia, spherocytosis, G6-PD

## CAUSES OF ACUTE AND CHRONIC BLOOD LOSS

(Perinatal: see p 15)
1. Epistaxis
2. Trauma
3. Ulceration: hiatus hernia, peptic ulcer, Meckel's diverticulum
4. Thrombocytopenia, e.g. idiopathic thrombocytopenia, leukaemia
5. Coagulation disorder, e.g. vitamin K deficiency, haemophilia

## CAUSES OF A LOW MEAN CORPUSCULAR VOLUME (MCV)

1. Iron deficiency anaemia
2. Thalassaemia trait - normal red cell count and normal mean corpuscular haemoglobin concentration (MCHC), *low* mean corpuscular haemoglobin (MCH)
3. Lead poisoning

## CAUSES OF PURPURA

Purpuric spots are capillary bleeds, which do not blanch on pressure, whereas erythema does.
   Due to vascular or platelet abnormality:

**Vascular**
1. Trauma, e.g. vigorous coughing, vomiting
2. Henoch-Schonlein (anaphylactoid) purpura
3. Meningococcaemia, bacterial endocarditis

**Thrombocytopenia**
($< 100 \times 10^9$/dl is highly significant)
1. Increased destruction: idiopathic thrombocytopenia
2. Consumption: shock, septicaemia
3. Decreased production: leukaemia, neuroblastoma

## CAUSES OF BRUISING

1. Trauma, accidental and non-accidental
2. Vascular (see above)
3. Platelets (see above)
4. Coagulation defects
    (i) Haemorrhagic disease of the newborn (vitamin K dependent factors - prothrombin, VII, IX, X)
   (ii) Consumption: shock, asphyxia, meningococcaemia
  (iii) Inherited: sex linked factor deficiencies VIII, IX = haemophilia (VIII), Christmas disease (IX)

# Oncology

## RELATIVE FREQUENCY OF CHILDHOOD MALIGNANCES

1. Acute lymphoblastic leukaemia (ALL)
2. Brain tumours
3. Lymphoma

## CAUSES OF HIGH WHITE CELL COUNT (WBC) (Lymphocytes excessively high)

1. Glandular fever, cytomegalovirus (both have atypical lymphocytes)
2. Pertussis (cough is obvious)
3. Still's disease (p 52) (may be difficult to differentiate clinically from leukaemia)
4. Leukaemia

## CONDITIONS PRESENTING LIKE LEUKAEMIA

1. Anaemia (see p 62)
2. Glandular fever
3. Oral infection, e.g. herpes stomatitis
4. Idiopathic thrombocytopenia
5. Bone pains from Still's disease, neuroblastoma

## CHARACTERISTICS OF CEREBRAL TUMOURS

Most (70%) are infratentorial in the posterior fossa and symptoms are those of:
1. Raised intracranial pressure, e.g. headache and vomiting
2. Ataxia due to cerebellar involvement. May be unilateral or bilateral depending on site of tumour
3. Cranial nerve palsies due to infiltration and as false localising signs from raised intracranial pressure (VIth cranial nerve)
4. Torticollis

Differential diagnosis of Wilms' tumour and abdominal neuroblastoma

|  | Wilms' tumour | Neuroblastoma |
| --- | --- | --- |
| Age (years) | < 5 | < 5 |
| Health | Well | Usually ill |
| Clinical | Swollen abdomen | Pale, weight loss and bone pain common |
| Mass | Lobulated, firm | Irregular edge, 'craggy' |
| Crosses midline | Rare | Common |
| Bilateral | Rare | Occasional |
| IVP pelvis | Grossly distorted | Pushed down, by mass above |
| Metastases (common sites) | Lungs | Bone (orbits) |

# Immunology, common infectious diseases and vaccinations

## NORMAL DEVELOPMENT OF IMMUNE SYSTEM

### Fetal
Immunoglobulins of G class pass from mother to baby and are not only responsible for protecting baby but also cause disease, e.g. rhesus incompatability

### Newborn
Maternal origin and levels of immunoglobulin G, (IgA and IgM low), falling progressively to very low level by 3 months.

Neutrophils are active but not yet good at fighting and thus babies are at increased risk of bacterial infection.

Lymphocyte function (B and T cell) not well developed, manifest by frequent superficial fungal (candida) infection and greater susceptibility to herpes simplex virus.

Thymus is large and easily seen on X ray (p 43). It shrinks rapidly in stress or cyanotic congenital heart disease

### Infant
Breast feeding protects via IgA, lactoferrin, interferon, lysozyme, maternal macrophages in the milk. Progressive rise in production of own immunoglobulins and cellular immunity

## CAUSES OF RECURRENT INFECTION

1. Normal development of immunity
2. Socioeconomic, and infants who are bottle fed (hygiene) or whose parents smoke
3. Secondary to disease:
   (i) Malnutrition
   (ii) Steroids, other drugs, i.e. side effect of treatment
   (iii) Underlying disorder, e.g. cystic fibrosis, sickle cell
   (iv) Structural abnormality, e.g. cleft palate and otitis media
4. Primary immune deficiency of immunoglobulins, white cells or complement systems

## SOME IMPORTANT INFECTIOUS DISEASES

| Disease | Incubation (days) | Characteristics and complications | Communicability |
|---|---|---|---|
| Chicken pox | 14 (7–21) | Vesicles spread down - face, trunk, proximal parts of limbs. Pneumonia, ataxia | −2 to +7 days from start of rash until spots crusted (dry) |
| Diphtheria | 3(1-6) | Grey-white membrane in nose, throat, 'toxic', myocarditis, bulbar palsy | 4 weeks or negative swabs ×2 |
| Enteric bacteria (salmonella, etc E.coli) | 3–23 | 3 major patterns: 1. diarrhoea 2. septicaemia 3. cholera like | Until asymptomatic and 3 negative stools |
| Fifth, or slapped cheek, disease | 4–14 | Bright red spots on cheeks, coalesce to look like a 'slap'; fine rash to body | 1 week, not apparent under 2 years old |
| Glandular fever | 14–56 | Sore throat, fever, lethargy; glands+++, hepatosplenomegaly, encephalitis, polyneuritis | 3 months, avoid salivary contact (cups, kissing) |
| Infectious hepatitis | 15–40 | Anicteric, itchy, anorexic; to icteric, pale stools, dark urine. Tender liver/ abdomen mimics appendicitis | 7 days minimum |
| Measles | 10(7–14) | 'Cold', photophobia, Koplik's spots, fever; then red rash, (face to trunk), conjunctivitis, otitis media, pneumonia. Encephalitis day 5–10 of illness | From 'cold' to 7 days after rash appears |
| Mumps | 17(14–28) | Fever, sore throat, pain on chewing, furred tongue, swollen parotid. Meningoencephalitis. Rarely orchitis, pancreatitis in children | −9 to +9 days after onset of swelling or when swelling goes |

| Disease | Incubation (days) | Characteristics and complications | Communicability |
|---------|-------------------|-----------------------------------|-----------------|
| Pertussis | 10(7–14) | Catarrhal for 1-2 weeks, then paroxysmal cough ± whoop 14–100 days. Recurs for up to 2 years. Death 1% <6 months old | 5 weeks from onset of cough |
| Polio | 14(7–21) | 'Cold', diarrhoea, muscle aches; after 7 days 'meningitic' and temperature rises again. Paralytic phase 3–7 days after onset of preparalytic meningitic phase. Spinal and bulbar forms | Until stool negative for virus, i.e. weeks |
| Roseola | | Fever for 3-4 days, as temperature falls rose-pink papules appear on trunk, neck, arms for a day | |
| Rubella | 17(14–19) | Mild 'cold', then rash (fine maculopapular), which fades from face as it spreads downwards, Thrombocytopenia 3 weeks later, arthritis in adolescence, congenital infection in pregnancy | 7 days from onset of rash |
| Scarlet fever | 2–5 | Tonsilitis, red spots on palate, strawberry tongue, red face with circum-oral pallor, fine red rash spreads to whole of body by 2–3 days, may then shed fine skin scales. Arthritis, nephritis | 3 days from start of penicillin |

## IMMUNISATION SCHEDULE

### Diphtheria-pertussis-tetanus (DPT) and oral polio

|  | No. of vaccinations |
|---|---|
| Start at 3–6 months | 1 |
| repeat 4–6 weeks later | 2 |
| then 4–6 months after 2nd | 3 |
| School entry: omit pertussis | 4 |
| School leaving: omit pertussis and diphtheria | 5 |

### Measles , mumps , rubella
1–2 years old

### BCG
10–13 years if Heaf test is negative

### Rubella
11–13 years for girls

## CONTRAINDICATIONS TO PERTUSSIS IMMUNISATION

### Absolute contraindications
1. Cerebral irritation in the neonatal period, fits at any time
2. Previous severe reaction to pertussis, not just local swelling, pain and slight fever

### Not absolute contraindication, but care in assessment
1. Parent or sibling has idiopathic epilepsy
2. Developmental delay with neurological cause
3. Neurological disease

### Postponement only
Acute febrile illness
   NB: Common parental misconceptions about contraindications include prematurity, heart disease and a family history of eczema or asthma

# Renal disorders

## COMMON FINDINGS

### Boys
1. Prepuce: retractile by 3 years in most boys, but, providing the opening is not scarred and there is no ballooning of the foreskin on micturition, not to be retractile is normal even in late childhood
2. Testes: in scrotum by 1 year, unless
   (i) absent bilaterally: consider intersex problems
   (ii) maldescended: after emerging from the superficial inguinal ring the testis goes ectopic, to the superficial inguinal pouch, femoral, perineal or public area. Torsion may occur
   (iii) undescended: normal line of descent, but arrested intra-abdominally, in the inguinal canal or high in the neck of the scrotum. Hernia common, fertility poor, malignancy more likely than in maldescent
   (iv) retractile: caused by cold hands or anxiety and descend if the child squats. If this manoeuvre fails, see (i) - (iii) above
3. Hydrocoeles: commoner in premature boys, gone by 1 year, transilluminate, and fingers can get above them, unlike inguinal hernias

### Girls
1. Perineum and vaginal mucosa pink prepubertally, darkening to becoming velvety red in puberty
2. Slight clear or white vaginal discharge is normal

## CAUSES OF FREQUENT MICTURITION

1. Physiological: age related
2. Emotional: stress, attention seeking
3. Urinary tract: infection, gross reflux, obstructive uropathy (e.g. neurogenic bladder, posterior urethral valves causing dribbling, poor stream)
4. Diabetes mellitus

## CAUSES OF POLYURIA

1. Psychological
2. Urinary tract infection
3. Diabetes mellitus and diabetes insipidus

## CAUSES OF ENURESIS
See p 27

## CAUSES OF COLOURED URINE

1. Dark yellow: concentrated (may cause red 'spot' of urates on napkin in boys and be mistaken for haematuria), bile
2. Pink to dark red: blood, food dyes, beeturia, drugs, e.g. danthron (Dorbanex)

## CAUSES OF HAEMATURIA
(may be microscopic)

1. Trauma to kidneys, renal tract
2. Urinary tract infection
3. Acute glomerulonephritis
4. Henoch-Schonlein (anaphylactoid) purpura
5. Recurrent haematuria syndrome occurring with fevers and upper respiratory tract infections
6. Wilms' tumour (rare)

## CAUSES OF ACUTE RENAL FAILURE BY AGE AT PRESENTATION

| Prerenal (pump failure, loss of fluid) | Renal | Postrenal (obstructive) |
|---|---|---|
| **Infants** | | |
| Acute D and V | UTI | Posterior |
| Septicaemia, congenital heart disease | Haemolytic – uraemic syndrome * | urethral valves |
| **Children** | | |
| Dehydration, trauma (acute blood loss), burns, scalds (protein loss) | Acute glomerulonephritis Acute tubular necrosis from prerenal cause | Neurogenic |

\* Haemolytic uraemic syndrome is uncommon, usually occurring in children under 1 year old, with infection, pallor, coma, fits; often hypertensive; may die.
   Laboratory findings: haemolytic anaemia, fragmented red cells, raised blood urea
D and V = diarrhoea and vomiting; UTI = urinary tract infection

## COMMON FEATURES OF ACUTE NEPHRITIS AND NEPHROTIC SYNDROME

|  |  | Nephritis | Nephrosis |
|---|---|---|---|
| Cause |  | Group AB H. streptococcus, Henoch-Schonlein, idiopathic | Unknown in 90% |
| Age (years) |  | 5–15, rarely preschool | Mainly preschool, up to 10 |
| Onset |  | Sudden | Days or weeks |
| Mode |  | Haematuria | Oedema |
| Temperature |  | Raised | Normal |
| BP |  | May be raised | Normal* |
| Urine | protein | ++/+++ | ++++ (Albustix) |
|  | blood | ++/+++ | Absent* |
|  | casts | Red cell | Hyaline/fatty |
| Plasma protein |  | Normal | Low albumin |
| Cholesterol |  | Normal | Raised |
| ASOT |  | Raised | Normal |
| C3 complement |  | Low | Normal |
| Prognosis |  | Good in 95% | Good unless raised blood urea/*BP,*haematuria; age < 1 or > 10 years |

## CAUSES OF RENAL MASSES

1. Unilateral cystic kidney, hydronephrosis, trauma, Wilms' tumour
2. Bilateral
   (i) hydronephrosis from obstruction
   (ii) cystic disease, infantile and adult forms
   (iii) tumour, e.g. Wilms,

## RENAL TUBULAR ACIDOSIS (RTA)

RTA is commonly due to a loss of bicarbonate from the proximal tubules, causing a metabolic acidosis. The Fanconi syndrome comprises RTA, glycosuria, aminoaciduria and excessive loss of phosphate and electrolytes, which is due to renal tubular damage secondary to lead poisoning or inborn errors of metabolism or is idiopathic with no known cause

# Metabolic disorders

## ACID-BASE DISORDERS

Infants have lower plasma concentrations of bicarbonate (18–24 mmol/1) than older children and adults, because the renal threshold is lower. They are therefore less able to acidify their urine and have less reserve (or defence) against acidosis

### Characteristics of acid-base disorders

|  | pH | $pCO_2$ | Base excess | Standard bicarbonate $(HCO_3^-)$ |
|---|---|---|---|---|
| Metabolic acidosis | down | down* | − n | down |
| Metabolic alkalosis | up | up* | + n | up |
| Respiratory acidosis | down | up | + n | up* |
| Respiratory alkalosis | up | down | − n | down* |

* After allowing time for compensation: quick respiratory (minutes), slow metabolic (hours).

n = Number of mmol/1 of acid (−) or alkali (+) to be corrected to achieve 'neutrality'

Correction of negative base excess (base deficit)
= body weight (kg) × base deficit × 0.3
= number of mmol alkali (sodium bicarbonate) needed

## IMPORTANT CAUSES OF ACID-BASE DISORDERS

1.  Metabolic acidosis
    (i)   Loss of bicarbonate: diarrhoea
    (ii)  Gain of strong acid: starvation, diabetes mellitus, shock, septicaemia, rarely renal failure and inborn errors of metabolism
2.  Metabolic alkalosis: pyloric stenosis
3.  Respiratory acidosis
    (i)   Central: depressed brain stem, e.g. drugs, infection
    (ii)  Obstructive: asthma, foreign body, epiglottitis

(iii)  Lung disease: respiratory distress syndrome (often a mixed respiratory and metabolic acidosis), cystic fibrosis
4.  Respiratory alkalosis: hysteria, encephalitis, early salicylate poisoning, compensatory for metabolic acidosis

*hyper-ventilation*

## HYPOCALCAEMIA

Normal values by age:
Newborn   <1.8 mmol/1 (may be lower in premature infants)
Older      <2.1 mmol/1

### Causes
1.  Rickets (p 30)
2.  Renal rickets
3.  Endocrine: Addison's disease, hypoparathyroidism
4.  Newborn: stress, cow's milk, maternal vitamin D deficiency

## CAUSES OF HYPOGLYCAEMIA

NB: Neonatal hypoglycaemia see p 16
1.  Malnutrition
2.  Fasting (previously called ketotic hypoglycaemia): usually 1–3 years old, thin, low birth weight
3.  Stress, e.g. septicaemia, hypothermia
4.  Alcohol
5.  Rare but important
    (i)  Reye's syndrome of hepatic failure, cerebral oedema with acidosis and hypoglycaemia after viral infection
    (ii)  Hypopituitarism
    (iii)  Hyperinsulinism

## INBORN ERRORS OF METABOLISM

Single enzyme deficiency, usually inherited as autosomal recessive (p 2), occasionally sex linked

## AMINOACIDURIA

Increased levels in both blood and urine in inborn error, e.g. phenylketonuria, or urine alone in renal tubular damage (p 73)

### Phenylketonuria
Deficiency of phenylalanine hydroxylase results in fair haired, blue eyed, eczematous children with mental retardation and fits. 'Mousey' smell. Guthrie test screens for raised phenylalanine blood level.
    Treatment: Diet low in phenylalanine, e.g. 'lofenalac' milk

**Maple syrup urine disease**
Deficiency of a branched chain decarboxylase causes high levels of leucine, isoleucine and valine, and urine smells like maple syrup (caramel). Within days or weeks of birth, vomiting, severe metabolic acidosis, seizures, hypoglycaemia, coma and death unless special diet given

# Orthopaedics

## NORMAL POSTURAL VARIATIONS

Neonate: Intrauterine position commonly causes postural deformities of feet (p 1)
Infant: Pigeon toe (metatarsus varus) is normal if passively correctable. Curly, overlapping toes usually self correct
Toddler: Flat feet and bow legs to 2 years
Preschool: Knock-knees, mild. More severe suggests rickets (p 30)

### Note
1. Asymmetry is always suspicious: consider congenital abnormality, trauma or tumour
2. Symmetrical deformity: endocrine, metabolic disorder is more likely

## SCREENING

### Congenital dislocation of the hip
1. Neonate (see p 9)
2. Infant
   a. One hip: shorter leg, limited abduction, extra skin fold, asymmetric buttock folds, 'telescoping' may be elicited (p 10). If walking, Trendelenburg dip present when taking weight on affected leg
   b. Bilateral: wide perineum, limited abduction, waddling walk

### Scoliosis
To exclude a postural curve the child should bend forward, arms hanging loosely down. If one shoulder is still higher than the other repeat forward flexion with child seated to eliminate asymmetry of leg length as the cause

## CAUSES OF SCOLIOSIS

1. Primary: postural, and infantile and adolescent types
2. Secondary
    (i) Bone: hemivertebrae
    (ii) Ligaments: Marfan's syndrome of tall stature, wide arm span, long digits, lens dislocation, aortic rupture, scoliosis. Autosomal dominant inheritance
    (iii) Muscle: muscular dystrophies
    (iv) Neurogenic: spina bifida, poliomyelitis, cerebral palsy

## CAUSES OF ACUTE PAINFUL JOINT OR LIMP

Remember, 'growing pains' and cramps are two common conditions with characteristic histories which must be differentiated from the following causes
1. Trauma
    (i) Severe
    (ii) Mild, may exacerbate slipped femoral epiphysis (see p 79)
    (iii) Non-accidental injury
2. Irritable hip
3. Infection: osteomyelitis especially *S. aureus, H. influenzae*, TB, viral, e.g. mumps, rubella
4. Henoch-Schonlein purpura (p 82)
5. Osteochondritis e.g. Perthe's disease of the hip
6. Haematological: Sickle cell disease, leukaemia
7. Rheumatic fever
8. Iatrogenic: drug reaction, serum sickness

## CAUSES OF CHRONIC ARTHRITIS

1. Infective: mycoplasma pneumoniae, brucellosis, TB
2. Postinfective: salmonella, shigella
3. Juvenile rheumatoid arthritis (JRA) or Still's disease
4. Chronic bowel disease: Crohn's, ulcerative colitis

## DIFFERENTIAL DIAGNOSIS OF STILL'S DISEASE, RHEUMATIC FEVER AND HENOCH-SCHONLEIN (ANAPHYLACTOID) PURPURA
See p 52

## DIFFERENTIAL DIAGNOSIS OF PATHOLOGY IN HIP, WITH PAIN IN HIP OR REFERRED TO KNEE

| | Age (years) | Clinical, and leg movement resisted | Investigations |
|---|---|---|---|
| 'Irritable hip' | 3–10 | Usually boy, well, internal rotation, abduction, extension | Normal |
| Septic hip | 0–5+ | Toxic, any movement pain++, (lies flexed adducted) | Blood culture +ive, X ray normal at first, WBC++; aspirate early |
| TB | 2–15 | Subacute, stiff and very painful | Hilar glands? Do Hb and WBC, ESR, Mantoux, urine for AAFB |
| Perthe's | 5–10 | Usually boy, well, abduction | X ray: loss of trabeculae, flattening of femoral head |
| Slipped epiphysis | 10–15 | Fat/very thin, well, internal rotation, abduction, extension | X ray: capital epiphysis falling back and downward in lateral view |

AAFB = acid and alcohol fast bacilli (tuberculosis)

# Dermatology

## COMMON SKIN CONDITIONS CAUSING DIAGNOSTIC CONFUSION

### Napkin dermatitis, intertrigo, seborrhoeic eczema and atopic eczema

| Age (months) | Cause | Clinical | Prognosis |
|---|---|---|---|
| 1–6 | **Napkin dermatitis** Prolonged skin contact with urine soaked nappy. Worse with faeces, may even cause ammonia burns | Groin folds spared, red, scald like or ulcers ('burns'), often infected | Good |
| 0.5–12 | **Intertrigo** Friction between folds of skin plus water/sweat | Fat babies, neck, axilla, groin; candida 'satellite' lesions common | Good |
| 0.5–3 | **Seborrhoea** Excess sebum production from sweat glands | Non-itchy, red skin and yellow greasy scales Spread: scalp, behind ears, neck, axillae; napkin area affected up to 8 months | Good |
| 3–24 | **Atopic eczema** Inherited | Itchy ++ Spread: scalp, face to extensor surfaces of the limbs; later to flexures. Strep. and staph. infections occur readily, occasionally *H. simplex* | Depends on age at onset: < 2 years = good > 2 years = poorer |

## Erythema

### Erythema nodosum
Raised red nodules over shins, rarely thighs, forearms
   Causes
   a. Unknown
   b. Infections: group A beta haemolytic streptococcus (BHS),
      viruses, TB
   c. Drugs, e.g. penicillin, sulphonamides

### Erythema multiforme
Wheals, red/purple target lesions, ulcers at mucocutaneous
junctions. If severe called Stevens-Johnson syndrome
   Causes
   a. Unknown
   b. Infection, e.g. *H. simplex*, *M. pneumoniae*
   c. Drugs, e.g. phenobarbitone

### Toxic erythema
Scarlet fever or measles like rash, followed by generalised peeling of
skin
   Causes
   a. BHS
   b. Drugs
   c. Unknown
(Differential diagnosis includes Kawasaki disease, characterised by
conjunctival injection, ulcers to oropharynx, swelling of hands and
feet, lymphadenopathy and cardiac involvement)

## DIFFERENTIAL DIAGNOSIS OF HENOCH-SCHONLEIN PURPURA (ANAPHYLACTOID) FROM IDIOPATHIC THROMBOCYTOPENIA (ITP)

| Age (years) | Cause | Clinical | Prognosis | Investigations |
|---|---|---|---|---|
| | | **Henoch-Schonlein** | | |
| 2–7 | β Haem. strep. Foods? Viral Unknown | 1. Oedema, erythema, purpura over extensor surfaces<br>2. Small joints swell<br>3. Colicky abdomen<br>4. Haematuria | Recurs for 7–10 weeks, for up to 2 years | Normal coagulation, normal capillary resistance |
| | | **ITP** | | |
| Any | Immune, occasionally rubella | Sudden onset, well, generalised purpura; bleeding from mouth, nose, haematuria, especially if becomes chronic (10% of cases) | Good in 90% | Platelets low, bleeding time prolonged |

# Management of common problems and emergencies

## AIRWAY/RESPIRATORY EMERGENCIES

### Acute epiglottitis
Symptoms of stridor, drooling, fever in a 3–7 year old who becomes toxic within a few hours, due to *H. influenzae* b found in throat and blood cultures. *Do not try to visualise the epiglottis* as this may precipitate a respiratory arrest

*Management*
Move to nearest intensive treatment unit (ITU). Intubation of airway by an experienced anaesthetist is likely to be needed. Humidified air/oxygen, chloramphenicol/ampicillin intravenously
  NB: Remember foreign body (FB) commonly, retropharyngeal abscess occasionally, diphtheria rarely may present in a similar way. See p 42 for comparison of FB, epiglottitis and laryngotracheo bronchitis

### Acute croup
Inspiratory stridor usually preceded by a few days' 'cold', though this is not always so and can easily appear like an epiglottitis. Age is 6 months to 3 years old, mild fever and constitutional upset. Wheeze common.

*Management*
Humidify air/oxygen, no antibiotic. Rarely is intubation necessary

### Acute respiratory failure

*Causes*
1. Central: head injury, drugs, convulsion, infection
2. Airway: acute epiglottitis, foreign body
3. Parenchymal: pneumonia, bronchiolitis, asthma
4. Chest wall: polio, trauma

*Clinical*
Restless, agitated from hypoxia, cyanosis, silent chest not moving sufficient air
   *Blood gases*: Low $PaO_2$ in oxygen (<8 kPa (55 mm Hg) in 40% $O_2$) and/or rising $CO_2$ in oxygen (>8 kPa in 80% $O_2$)

*Management*
Secure airway, bag and mask, intubate, assist ventilation. Deal with primary cause

**Acute bronchiolitis**
'Cold' is followed, 3–5 days later, by progressive cough, wheeze, difficulty in feeding, signs as for asthma (below), often fine inspiratory crepitations, in infant 6 weeks to 6 months old; due to respiratory syncitial virus (RSV)

*Management*
1. Oxygen
2. Suction of secretions
3. Tube feeding or i.v. fluids if unable to feed orally
4. Antibiotics may be given according to age and severity of the illness, usually because bacterial infection is suspected

May recur. One third later develop asthma

**Acute asthma**
From 1 year old, expiratory wheeze, difficulty in speaking, head extended, nostrils flared, chest increased anteroposterior diameter, accessory muscles working, rapid pulse, may have pulsus paradoxus (pulse weaker on inspiration), cyanosis in air

*Management*
1. Nebulised sympathomimetic, e.g. salbutamol, to be repeated according to response
2. Oxygen, before 1 if hypoxic/cyanosed, or via nebuliser
3. Theophylline i.v., not by rectal suppository, and less than full dose if already on oral treatment
4. Consider continuous infusion of i.v. fluid, theophylline and hydrocortisone if inadequate response; introduce oral prednisolone and bronchodilators as soon as practicable
5. Antibiotics only if good evidence of infection. Monitor pulse, respiration; chest *x* ray and blood gases in severe or deteriorating episode

**Pneumonia**
Bronchopneumonia commoner then lobar pneumonia, especially in the preschool child

*Causes*
Primary viral or bacterial (p 41) or secondary, e.g. post measles, whooping cough, milk inhalation, etc.

Babies may be very ill, grey, cyanosed, respiratory rate and effort increased, and the episode complicated by a febrile convulsion.

In older children lobar pneumonia can mimic acute appendicitis, and meningism may suggest meningitis. Upper respiratory 'rattle' due to secretions not to be confused with fine crackles from parenchymal fluid, or the coarse crackles from fluid/secretions in bronchi

*Investigations*
Chest x ray (see pp. 43–46), Hb and WBC, throat swab, blood culture, Mantoux, according to severity. If episodes recur consider sweat test (after the first if staphylococcal), look for foreign body or immune deficiency

*Management*
Suck out secretions from the airway, give physiotherapy, oxygen and nasogastric or i.v. feeds according to need. Antibiotics in clinical favour include ampicillin, or gentamicin and penicillin in sick infants. Flucloxacillin is added to ampicillin if staphylococcal pneumonia is suspected

## CARDIAC EMERGENCIES

### Cardiac failure

*Symptoms to note*
Lethargy, feeding problems or breathless on feeding, sweating, failure to thrive, recent excessive weight gain or oedema, blue attacks. Often seems precipitated or exacerbated by an intercurrent illness, e.g. pneumonia

*Signs*
Rapid pulse and respiration, hepatomegaly. Check femoral pulses and BP (see p 47) for heart sounds, etc)

*Investigations*
Chest x ray, ECG, Hb, WBC, E and U, bacteriology

*Management*
1. Diuretic, e.g. frusemide, check electrolytes and urea regularly at first, consider potassium supplements unless spironolactone added
2. Digoxin (may be omitted or relatively contraindicated, e.g. Fallot's tetralogy). Oral administration is almost always sufficient.

Maintenance is 1/4 loading dose. Check pulse rate before each
dose. If slow or bigemenous, omit dose
3. Oxygen
4. Morphine for agitation
5. Position: sitting or on an incline, head up
6. Treat precipitating event, i.e. anaemia or infection
    Monitor weight, pulse, respirations, liver size

**Cardiorespiratory arrest**
Remember 'A-B-C-D-E'

*Airway*
Clear muck with swab round finger/suction. (Meconium in newborn
should be aspirated as head is delivered; if fresh, intubate and apply
suction with wide bore catheter to mouth or suction direct to end of
endotracheal tube. Chest is constricted by encircling with hands to
prevent breathing until meconium removed)

*Breath*
Baby's nose and mouth covered in mouth to mouth, older children
mouth only. Give breath according to size, ensuring the chest moves
with each breath. Bag and mask: use plastic airway, be sure mask
seal on face is tight, support jaw

*Cardiac output*
Failure of pump or blood volume
Pump:              1. Neonate, use 2 fingers on mid-sternum
                   2. <1 year old, circle chest with hands, thumbs
                      pressing down on mid-sternum
                   3. >1 year old, use heel of hand on mid- to lower
                      sternum
Rate:              1 breath to 5 compressions at 80–100 compressions
                   per minute
Effectiveness:     carotid/femoral pulse felt
Blood volume:      plasma expander or 0.9% saline
                   20 ml/kg in hypovolaemic shock

*Drugs*
A-B-C-D:  Adrenaline/atropine/antidote (e.g. naloxone in the
          newborn)
          Bicarbonate
          Calcium salts
          Dextrose

*Electrocardiograph*
Electrocardiograph for arrhythmias
    NB: Continue attempts beyond half an hour even if no heart beat if
hypothermia from cold water immersion, or drug ingestion
suspected

## BURNS AND SCALDS

### Immediate action in the home
1. Scald: strip off affected clothing, as it retains the hot liquid
2. Scald/burn: if small immerse in cold running water, or add ice to a basin of cold water, until cool. Cover area in a clean dry sheet, towel or dressing

### Hospital assessment
1. Airway (respiratory tract burn likely if soot in nostrils, or wheezy)
2. Appropriate analgesia, e.g. morphine i.v.
3. Plasma expanders if >10% of surface affected, to prevent shock, renal failure. Colloid (plasma/plasma protein fraction/Haemaccel) or Ringer's solution. Blood in full thickness (FT) burn/scald
4. Weigh
5. Hb check for early haemoconcentration, and subsequent anaemia in full thickness burn
6. Monitor urine output, blood and urine biochemistry, beware of renal failure

   NB: Rule of 9s does not apply, e.g. infant head 18%, legs 13%, arms 9%, trunk 18% front/back.
   Remember full thickness is anaesthetic to pin prick.
   Consider non-accidental injury, especially in preschool child

## OTHER ACUTE INFECTIONS

### Acute diarrhoea
Diarrhoea constitutes an increase in frequency and fluid content of stools

*Clinical signs*
Clinical signs of isotonic dehydration as a percentage loss of body weight:
5% (mild = 50 ml/kg): lethargic, loss of skin turgor, dry mouth, fontanelle slack
10% (moderate = 100 ml/kg): also tachycardia, tachypnoea, fontanelle and eyes sunken, mottled skin, oliguria
15% (severe = 150 ml/kg): also shock, coma, hypotension
   Symptoms occur earlier in hypotonic dehydration (serum sodium <130 mmol/l), later in hypernatraemic (>150 mmol/l) dehydration.

*Investigations*
In all but mild cases, do Hb, WBC, E and U, bacteriology of stool (x3), throat, urine and blood
1. Oral or nasogastric feeds unless unconscious, absent bowel sounds, 10% or more dehydrated or shocked. In shock give

plasma or 0.9% saline i.v. 20 ml/kg over 20 minutes. If i.v. fluids are needed give 4% dextrose/0.18% saline for 24 hours. Bicarbonate may be given if acidosis is severe, but care is needed (see diabetic ketoacidosis)
2. Fluid replacement = percentage dehydration (above) plus maintenance (150 ml/kg in infants, 50–100 ml/kg in children) plus ongoing losses from vomiting or diarrhoea
3. Oral rehydration solution (ORS) recommended by the World Health Organization (WHO) for developing countries contains sodium 90 mmol/l, potassium 30 mmol/l, bicarbonate 30 mmol/l, chloride 90 mmol/l and glucose 2% (110 mmol/l). Developed countries still prefer an ORS with lower sodium (30–50 mmol/l) and often a higher sugar content (4%), e.g. Diorylate
4. Administer ORS little and often (5–10 ml every 1–5 minutes is WHO policy) to replace deficit in 6 hours, offering extra after each vomit or diarrhoea. Breast feeding should continue. Water may be offered after the diarrhoea has eased, or in a ratio of 2 ORS:1 water during rehydration
5. Reintroduce diluted whole/powdered cow's milk over 1–3 days, starches (potato, rice) within 1–2 days. Soy milk may be preferred for a few days to avoid the post enteritis (usually transient), lactose and cow's milk intolerance
6. Hypernatraemic dehydration. The deficit is corrected more slowly, over 24–72 hours to avoid convulsions.
   Monitor urine output for signs of renal failure, weigh regularly, investigate blood biochemistry and gases as required

## Meningitis, acute bacterial
Initial signs may be non-specific in the infant, e.g. initially presenting as gastroenteritis. Irritable cry, coma, convulsion, apnoea, signs of a bulging fontanelle, head retraction and resistance to flexion. (Meningism is a feature of respiratory infections, but lumbar puncture (LP) must be considered).
   Associated conditions are common, e.g. otitis media and purpura in meningococcal infection. Onset is rapid in the neonate, and in pneumococcal or meningococcal infection, and is often preceded by a 'cold' for some days before if H. influenzae

### Investigations
CSF cells, Gram stain and glucose, bacteriology, Hb, WBC, E and U, blood glucose, chest x ray

### Diagnosis
CSF turbid, polymorphs >20/mm³, protein >0.45 g/l, glucose <2/3 blood glucose

*Treatment*
Initially, until culture and sensitivities are known:
   Neonate: *E. coli* and group B haemolytic streptococcus likely,
therefore a newer cephalosporin or chloramphenicol is given with
benzyl penicillin. Treat for 3 weeks
   After 3 months old: *H. influenzae*, meningococcus and
pneumococcus likely, therefore ampicillin in high dose often with
chloramphenicol in case *H. influenzae* is resistant. Treat for 10 days

*Important complications*
1. Convulsions
2. Cerebral oedema, subdural effusion, hydrocephalus
3. Hyponatraemia from inappropriate antidiuretic hormone release
4. Deafness: always screen hearing immediately on recovery
5. Drug fever: rise of fever after initial fall
6. Long term: mental handicap, cerebral palsy, epilepsy, deaf

**Osteomyelitis/septic arthritis**
Reluctance to use a limb, local swelling or tenderness may progress
to a 'toxic' looking septicaemic infant or child. The hip is usually
involved in osteomyelitis of the femur in infancy, so early diagnosis
and treatment are vital in preventing damage to the femoral head

*Investigations*
Blood culture, Hb, WBC, x rays

*Treatment*
Intravenous antibiotics, in expectation of a penicillinase producing
*Staphylococcus aureus* (70% of cases). Flucloxacillin plus ampicillin
is a popular combination. Immobilise the limb, watch.
   Surgery is indicated immediately in septic hip in infants and, if
poor response to treatment after 24 hours, in older children

**Urinary tract infection**

*Clinical*
1. Neonate: poor feeding, vomiting, fever, weight loss, conjugated
   jaundice, boys>girls
2. Preschool: vomiting, diarrhoea, failure to thrive, irritability and
   crying, fever, girls<boys
3. School age: localisation of pain to suprapubic or loin area, fever,
   polydipsia, polyuria, dysuria
   NB: Dysuria is also a symptom of vulvitis or balinitis in the older
child and as likely as UTI if otherwise asymptomatic, but this is
diagnosed *only* after appropriate investigation as the consequence
of untreated UTI may be renal scarring

*Investigations*
Always check blood pressure, Hb, WBC, E and U, serum creatinine, urine ± blood culture (septicaemic?), ultrasound to look for calyceal dilatation from infection or obstruction of ureters, kidney *x* ray and radio isotope studies for scarring, pelvi-ureteric obstruction and ureteral reflux, duplex collecting systems, bladder diverticuli/obstruction

*Bacteriology*
< 1 year old = *E. coli*
> 1 year old = 1/3 each *E. coli*, proteus, others
Significance of colony counts in the diagnosis of UTI:
a. $10^5$/ml or more in a clean catch (CCU) or midstream urine (MSU), in at least 2 separate samples
b. $10^4$/ml via catheter
c. *any* growth on suprapubic urine (SPU) obtained by bladder puncture
d. only *no* growth in a single bag urine (contamination so likely, do CCU/MSU/SPU for confirmatory *proof* of infection)
Pus cells in urine: may be *absent* in urinary
   infection, yet up to 100/mm$^3$ in girl's bag urine, or more if vulvitis or balinitis is present. Treat according to antibiotic sensitivities, give i.v. gentamycin + ampicillin if septicaemic, fluids ++

## MISCELLANEOUS PROBLEMS

### Diabetic ketoacidosis
Polydipsia, polyuria for days or weeks only. Weight loss, dehydration, vomiting, abdominal pain ('appendicitis?'), deep breaths ('pneumonia', 'uraemia'?), infection associated, e.g. urinary infection or 'thrush', coma ('hypoglycaemia'?) Check weight, assess dehydration

*Investigations*
Blood glucose, blood gases, E and U, Hb and WBC, bacteriology

*Management*

*Severe ketoacidosis*
1. Rehydrate using 0.9% saline. Requirement = per cent dehydration (10% = 100 ml/kg) plus maintenance (50–100 ml/kg) intravenously, adding potassium as urine flow recommences and biochemistry indicates
2. Insulin, soluble. Initial bolus 0.1–0.5 U/kg, then i.v. infusion or hourly i.m. injections (0.1 U/kg/hour) until blood glucose falls to 15 mmol/l, when 4% glucose/0.18% saline infusion replaces 0.9% saline, and soluble insulin is then given every 4–6 hours
3. Bicarbonate is now rarely given because $HCO_3 \rightleftharpoons HO^- + CO_2$, and

CO$_2$ crosses into the brain, CO$_2$ + H$_2$O $\rightleftharpoons$ H$_2$CO$_3$ i.e. acid rises in the brain, delaying recovery of consciousness. Monitor input, output and biochemistry carefully

*Mild to moderate ketoacidosis, or in recovery phase from severe*
1. Insulin, soluble 0.5 U/kg subcutaneously before each main meal, until blood glucose <15 mmol/l and no more ketonuria. Urine tests for glucose can be used in a sliding scale. Now consider long term insulin. Soluble twice daily in 0–3 year olds, 1 or 2 injections of medium acting insulin in middle childhood, and 2 of soluble plus medium acting insulin in adolescence. Timing – before breakfast and main evening meal
2. Diet. Total calories = 1000 plus 100 per year of life, half as carbohydrate in 10 g 'exchanges' for main meals and snacks between to avoid hypoglycaemia. Avoid extra fat (one third of calories). High fibre foods are currently encouraged for their slower release of carbohydrates and hence less wide and wild excursions of the blood glucose than with refined foods

## Hypoglycaemia

*Definition*
This is related to age (see p 16, 75)

*Signs*
The usual signs of hypoglycaemia are similar to those in adults. The young child, however, may become drowsy or merely seem more difficult than usual! The presence of ketones on the breath or urine without hyperglycaemia/glycosuria is a sign of fasting hypoglycaemia (ketotic hypoglycaemia), to which some small for age preschool children are prone (p 75).
   Be wary of hypoglycaemia after ethyl alcohol ingestion in children

*Investigation*
Blood glucose, and insulin level if persistently low blood glucose despite adequate treatment. Inappropriately high insulin for the low blood glucose indicates hyperinsulinism (excess production by pancreas/non-accidental administration)

*Management*
Oral glucose if able, otherwise i.v. glucose 0.5 g/kg body weight as 50% solution

## Poisoning

*Immediate action in the home*
EXCEPT with volatile hydrocarbons or caustics or when child is unconscious, induce vomiting with fingers, *not* salt water, etc

*Hospital assessment*
1. Establish a poison(s) has been taken, its name, amount, when, how. Consider non-accidental ingestion. Check with a National Poisons Information Service centre
2. Induce vomiting with syrup of ipecac, 15 ml + glass of water, within 6 hours of ingestion, up to 24 hours for salicylates. Repeat after 20 minutes if no result. Contraindicated in caustic, petrol or white spirit ingestion. Gastric lavage for the unconscious, with protected airway
3. Specific antidotes
   Acetyl cysteine/methionine, for paracetamol poisoning
   Activated charcoal for tricyclics, opiates or slow release theophylline poisoning
   Alkali diuresis for salicylate or phenobarbitone poisoning
   Desferrioxamine for iron
   Fuller's Earth for paraquat
   Glucose for alcohol (hypoglycaemia may be severe)
   Naloxone for Lomotil, opiates
   Oxygen for carbon monoxide poisoning
4. General measures: observation and, where appropriate, close monitoring of airway, circulation, temperature, fluid balance, blood glucose

## Pyrexia

A frequent presentation at all ages; most episodes are due to viral infection. Absence of localising signs, at least initially, is common. Always consider contacts, foreign travel even up to a year ago (e.g. malaria), environmental hazards (pets, untreated milk, etc).

Investigations in the acutely ill: bacterial 'screen' i.e. throat swab, stool, blood culture, urine. Lumbar puncture may be necessary. Hb, WBC, chest x ray and Mantoux (thick film for malaria, serology for typhoid, hepatitis, glandular fever, etc, in appropriate cases). The ESR is often high in acute viral or bacterial infections as well as in more chronic illness such as TB, subacute bacterial endocarditis, collagenoses, malignancy, etc.

In practice an 'infection screen' and blood culture, Hb, WBC and ESR, chest x ray and Mantoux are done, followed by a period of observation. Only then are further tests likely to be helpful

## Seizures

The most common cause is a febrile convulsion. In the absence of fever, epilepsy must be considered. Status epilepticus is a fit lasting more than 30 minutes or several fits with failure to regain consciousness between them.

*Action*
1. Move child away from danger, e.g. heater. Place prone to avoid inhalation of vomit or saliva
2. Loosen clothing round the neck, do not attempt to prise open the mouth as teeth may be broken and inhaled and the tongue pushed back, occluding the airway
3. Give diazepam i. v., 1 + 1 mg for each year of life or as rectal preparation, e.g. Stesolid (1–3 years give 5 mg; 10 mg for older children). If no response after 10 minutes give paraldehyde 1 ml for each year of life, in divided dose if more than 2 ml, deep into each buttock. Phenytoin i. v. is an alternative or additional drug if fits continue
4. Continuing seizure/duration longer than 30 minutes is an indication for general anaesthesia
5. Restrict fluids and consider mannitol and dexamethasone to combat potential cerebral oedema. If febrile, undress, tepid sponge, give antipyretic
6. Oral drugs may be indicated, both short and long term

*Investigations*
Blood glucose (Dextrostix/BM stix), especially during a prolonged fit. Lumbar puncture in first febrile convulsions under 2 years old, prolonged or focal and if meningism present. Others by suspected cause (p 25), e.g. skull and chest X ray, E and U, serum calcium, Hb and WBC, EEG

*Some types of seizure requiring specific treatment*
1. Infantile spasms: ACTH injections or corticosteroids, and a benzodiazepine, e.g. nitrazepam
2. Petit mal: ethosuximide or valproate
3. Temporal lobe or focal epilepsy: carbemazepine or phenytoin

## Sudden infant death syndrome (SIDS)

*Incidence*
1–2 per 1000 in Britain

*Definition*
Sudden and unexpected death after which a properly performed autopsy fails to reveal a major cause of death. Predominantly 1 month to 1 year old, an apparently normal baby dies. Commoner in boys, of low birth weight, in winter, in adverse social and domestic conditions. Recent weight loss and hyperpyrexia are at present implicated in the apparently spontaneous final apnoea. Some authors also implicate a poor appreciation of symptoms in babies by medical attendants and parents

*Action*
1. Resuscitation may be appropriate
2. If the history and examination do not suggest prior illness or injury and suspicion of the parents seems unfounded, they should be told cot death (SIDS) is likely
3. The Coroner's (Procurator Fiscal in Scotland) duty to investigate is explained together with the need for an autopsy and the role of the police, who will ask for a statement and possibly for identification of the body and may visit the home and remove bedding for examination
4. Emphasis is placed on the routine nature of the inquiries and the absence of a desire to blame parents or the person caring for the victim
5. Parents may wish to hold their baby, and this should be suggested
6. Inform family doctor, health visitor and social services (if involved already)
7. Suppress lactation if breast feeding

**Suspected non-accidental injury (NAI)**
Where abuse is or was inflicted or knowingly not prevented by person(s) caring for a child *and* signs are present of physical injury and/or neglect, drug administration, failure to thrive, emotional or sexual abuse

*Assessment*
1. Injuries inconsistent with explanation, delay in seeking help, medical advice sought for repeated minor injuries
2. Parent young, single, mentally ill, know to social services, low IQ (though remember anyone can be an abusing parent!)
3. Child separated at some time in infancy, child handicapped
4. Physically appears neglected, withdrawn or drugged, bruising of differing ages or bilateral black eyes, scalds or burns, old and new fractures, internal injuries e.g. subdurals, torn frenulum in mouth, retinal detachment and bleeds, torn abdominal organ, bruising of genitals

*Investigations*
Photographs, skeletal survey, coagulation studies, venereological/ forensic tests

*Action*
1. Notify senior medical and social work staff immediately
2. Until the child is in a place of safety or security is assured confrontation is best avoided, and then should be undertaken only by experienced staff

3. If removal seems likely seek a Place of Safety Order via social workers or NSPCC. The police do not need a magistrate's order (useful in an emergency!)

4. Case conference to be called at the earliest possible time to:
   (i) Establish what has taken place: is it NAI?
   (ii) Consider immediate action to protect the child (whether to return home, remain in a place of safety, take out a Place of Safety Order if not yet obtained, or institute Care Proceedings in the Magistrates Court)
   (iii) What further information, investigations and procedures may be necessary to make plans for the child's future
   (iv) Should the name of the child, siblings or other children in the household be placed on the 'At risk' register?
   (v) Name a coordinator, the 'key worker', and the 'prime worker', who works with the family (may be the same person)

# Abbreviations

| | |
|---|---|
| ABO | Refers to the major blood groups A, B and O |
| D and V | Diarrhoea and vomiting |
| E and U | Electrolytes and urea (in serum or plasma, includes sodium, potassium, chloride, bicarbonate and urea) |
| ECG | Electrocardiogram |
| EEG | Electroencephalogram |
| ESR | Erythrocyte sedimentation rate |
| G6-PD | Glucose 6-phosphate dehydrogenase |
| Hb | Haemoglobin |
| i.v. | Intravenous |
| PR | Time interval between beginning of the P wave and the R wave on an electrocardiograph (ECG) |
| TB | Tuberculosis |
| TORCH | Congenital infections: Toxoplasmosis, Other e.g. syphilis Rubella, Cytomegalovirus, *Herpes simplex* |
| UTI | Urinary tract infection |
| WBC | White blood cell count |

# Index